T0226617

Diabetes

Editor

CELIA M. LEVESQUE

CRITICAL CARE NURSING CLINICS OF NORTH AMERICA

www.ccnursing.theclinics.com

Consulting Editor
JAN FOSTER

March 2013 • Volume 25 • Number 1

ELSEVIER

Elsevier Inc., 1600 John F. Kennedy Blvd., Suite 1800, Philadelphia, PA 19103-2899

http://www.theclinics.com

CRITICAL CARE NURSING CLINICS OF NORTH AMERICA Volume 25, Number 1
March 2013 ISSN 0899-5885, ISBN-13: 978-1-4557-7077-9

Editor: Katie Saunders
Developmental Editor: Nicole Congleton

Critical Care Nursing Clinics of North America (ISSN 0899-5885) is published quarterly by Elsevier Inc., 360 Park Avenue South, New York, NY 10010-1710. Months of issue are March, June, September, and December. Business and Editorial Offices: 1600 John F. Kennedy Blvd., Suite 1800, Philadelphia, PA 19103-2899. Periodicals postage paid at New York, NY and additional mailing offices. Subscription prices are $144.00 per year for US individuals, $308.00 per year for US institutions, $76.00 per year for US students and residents, $192.00 per year for Canadian individuals, $385.00 per year for Canadian institutions, $219.00 per year for international individuals, $385.00 per year for international institutions and $111.00 per year for Canadian and foreign students/residents. To receive student/resident rate, orders must be accompanied by name of affiliated institution, data of term, and the signature of program/residency coordinator on institution letterhead. Orders will be billed at individual rate until proof of status is received. Foreign air speed delivery is included in all Clinics subscription prices. All prices are subject to change without notice. **POSTMASTER:** Send address changes to Critical Care Nursing Clinics of North America, Elsevier Health Sciences Division, Subscription Customer Service, 3251 Riverport Lane, Maryland Heights, MO 63043. **Customer Service: 1-800-654-2452 (US and Canada); 314-447-8871 (outside US and Canada). Fax: 314-447-8029. E-mail: JournalsCustomerService-usa@elsevier.com (for print support) and JournalsOnlineSupport-usa@elsevier.com (for online support).**

Reprints. For copies of 100 or more of articles in this publication, please contact the Commercial Reprints Department, Elsevier Inc., 360 Park Avenue South, New York, New York, 10010-1710; Tel.: (212) 633-3813, Fax: (212) 462-1935, and E-mail: reprints@elsevier.com.

Critical Care Nursing Clinics of North America is covered in MEDLINE/PubMed (Index Medicus), International Nursing Index, Nursing Citation Index, Cumulative Index to Nursing and Allied Health Literature, and RNdex Top 100.

Printed and bound by CPI Group (UK) Ltd, Croydon, CR0 4YY

Transferred to digital print 2012

Contributors

CONSULTING EDITOR

JAN FOSTER, PhD, RN, CNS
College of Nursing, Texas Woman's University, Houston, Texas

EDITOR

CELIA M. LEVESQUE, RN, MSN, NP-C, CNS-BC, BC-ADM, CDE
Department of Endocrine Neoplasia and Hormonal Disorders, The University of Texas MD Anderson Cancer Center, Houston, Texas

AUTHORS

ASHRAF ABBAS, RN, MSN, ACNP-BC
Vascular Surgery Service, Michael E. DeBakey Veterans Affairs Medical Center, Houston, Texas

VERONICA BRADY, MSN, FNP-BC, BC-ADM, CDE
Department of Endocrine Neoplasia and Hormonal Disorders, The University of Texas MD Anderson Cancer Center, Houston, Texas

BECKY CHILDERS, RN, MSNspEd, CDE
Director of Joslin Diabetes Center Affiliate at St. Joseph Medical Center and Advanced Wound Care, St. Joseph Medical Center, Houston, Texas

KATE CRAWFORD, RN, MSN, ANP-C, BC-ADM
Department of Endocrine Neoplasia and Hormonal Disorders, The University of Texas MD Anderson Cancer Center, Houston, Texas

ESPERANZA GALVAN, MS, RN, CVRN, CDE
Manager, CardioPulmonary Management Program, Harris Health System, Houston, Texas

LINDA WILLS GIBSON, RN, MSN, CRRN, ANP-C
Director of PAVE Clinic (Prevention of Amputation for Veterans Everywhere), Rehabilitation Care Line, Michael E. DeBakey Veterans Affairs Medical Center, Houston, Texas

TALAR L. GLOVER, MS, RN, CNS, CDE
Director, Diabetes Service Line and Patient Education, Harris Health System, Houston, Texas

JUDY KEAVENY, RN, MSN, CNS M-S, CDE
Department of General Internal Medicine, The University of Texas MD Anderson Cancer Center, Houston, Texas

CORI KOPECKY, MSN, RN, OCN
Clinical Nurse, The University of Texas MD Anderson Cancer Center, Houston, Texas

CELIA M. LEVESQUE, RN, MSN, NP-C, CNS-BC, BC-ADM, CDE
Department of Endocrine Neoplasia and Hormonal Disorders, The University of Texas MD Anderson Cancer Center, Houston, Texas

ASHLEY MARTIN, MSN, RN, ANP-BC
Department of Endocrine Neoplasia and Hormonal Disorders, MD Anderson Cancer Center, Houston, Texas

DEBORAH MCCREA, RN, MSN, CNS, CEN, CFRN, EMT-P
Professor, Department of Emergency Medical Services, Houston Community College, Houston, Texas

JOHNNY L. ROLLINS, RN, MSN, ANP-C
Department of Endocrine Neoplasia and Hormonal Disorders, The University of Texas MD Anderson Cancer Center, Houston, Texas

BARB SCHREINER, PhD, RN, CDE, BC-ADM, CPLP
Core Faculty Professor, Department of Nursing, Capella University, Minneapolis, Minnesota

Contents

hypoglycemia, diabetic ketoacidosis, hyperosmolar hyperglycemic state, dehydration, and electrolyte imbalances. Many factors influence the optimal care plan, including the usual home diabetes regimen, the level of diabetes control before surgery, the surgery type, the duration of surgery, and the amount of time the patient will be fasting. An optimal plan of care is based on a thorough presurgical assessment and prescribing a regimen that will minimize acute complications. This article discusses recommendations for target blood glucose and diabetes medication adjustment during the perioperative period.

Hyperglycemia after solid organ transplantation increases the risk for wound infection, poor healing time, graft rejection, and graft loss. In patients without a history of diabetes, uncontrolled hyperglycemia increases the risk for advancement to diabetes mellitus. Controlling hyperglycemia can reduce the prevalence of new-onset diabetes after transplantation. This article discusses the current literature concerning blood glucose management after solid organ transplantation, the issues surrounding hyperglycemia in the patient with a solid organ transplant, and how to manage hyperglycemia after solid organ transplant.

Noninsulin antidiabetic medications coupled with diet and exercise are effective in managing most patients with type 2 diabetes. However, it is essential to evaluate the safety and effectiveness of the home antidiabetic medication regimen when the patient is hospitalized. Prescribers need to be aware of the mechanism of action of each class, contraindications, precautions, and adverse effects to formulate a safe and effective management plan. This article details the different classes of noninsulin antidiabetic medications, the mechanism of action, metabolism, elimination, dose form, usual and maximum doses, contraindications, precautions, common adverse reactions, and implications for use in the hospitalized patient.

Hyperglycemia is common and often unrecognized among hospitalized patients, and it increases the risk of poor outcome, increased length of stay, and increased cost. Hyperglycemia can complicate features of underlying disease and some therapies. This article discusses physiology and types of diabetes, glycemic targets in the noncritical care setting, factors that contribute to hyperglycemia and hypoglycemia in the hospitalized patient, insulin types, common insulin regimens used in the hospital setting, and implications for the nurse.

Mortality from cardiovascular disease is 2 to 4 times higher in patients with type 2 diabetes compared with patients with similar demographic characteristics but without diabetes. The management of hypertension in patients with diabetes is as important as glucose control in the prevention of long-term diabetes complications. This article discusses the incidence of hypertension in diabetes, the impact of hypertension on the development of long-term complications, diagnosis of hypertension in patients with diabetes, blood pressure goals, the treatment of hypertension in patients with diabetes, and antihypertension medications.

Heart failure affects more than five million Americans. It is a health and financial burden on the US health care system. The 5-year mortality of heart failure with diabetes is about 50%. This article discusses the treatment of heart failure in the patient with diabetes, including developing effective communication skills between physicians and nurses, developing an effective plan for transitioning the patient between care settings, documenting patient visits consistently and clearly, and performing medication reconciliation at each visit. This article also discusses the need for monitoring readmission for heart failure, length of stay, discharge on beta-blocker, and vaccination rate.

When a child is diagnosed with diabetes and admitted to the pediatric intensive care unit for metabolic stabilization, there is little time to provide survival skills and education, much less support the family through the impact of the diagnosis. Yet, critical care nurses can begin the family's adaptation and recovery. This article explores the educational and support needs of the newly diagnosed child and the child who is admitted repeatedly. A model of survival topics is presented and the role of the critical care nurse is emphasized with tips for returning the family to a new normal.

More than 375,000 Americans manage their diabetes with an insulin pump, and this number continues to increase. Many of these patients will want to remain on their insulin pump while hospitalized, so the nurse needs to know about how to care for the hospitalized patient wearing an insulin pump. This article discusses the benefits of intensive insulin therapy, how the insulin pump works, initial insulin-pump dosing, candidate selection, advantages and disadvantages of using an insulin pump, troubleshooting the pump, nursing care of the hospitalized patient wearing an

CRITICAL CARE NURSING
CLINICS OF NORTH AMERICA

NOW AVAILABLE FOR YOUR iPhone and iPad

Preface

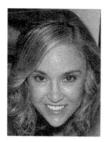

Celia M. Levesque, RN, MSN, NP-C, CNS-BC, BC-ADM, CDE
Editor

Diabetes mellitus affects 8.3% of the US population. People with diabetes are twice as likely to be hospitalized, and their length of stay is approximately 30% longer compared to patients without diabetes. The management of blood glucose and the complications of hyperglycemia in the hospitalized patient with and without diabetes are the subject of many research studies. This issue covers the current guidelines for management of diabetes and hyperglycemia in the hospitalized patient. The issue begins with a review of the general recommendations for hospitalized patients with diabetes and hyperglycemia by Crawford. Brady then discusses the management of hyperglycemia and diabetes for patients in the intensive care unit. Martin discusses indications and adjustment of an insulin drip as well as commonly used drips. Perioperative management of diabetes and hyperglycemia, discussed by Levesque, can be complicated and is crucial for the prevention of acute complications and the reduction of the risk for morbidity and mortality. The use of steroids in transplant patients commonly causes hyperglycemia in those without diabetes and uncontrolled diabetes in those with diabetes. Rollins discusses the management in patients after solid organ transplantation. The use of noninsulin diabetes medications in hospitalized patients is discussed by Kopecky. The use of insulin and commonly used insulin regimens in patients who are not critically ill are discussed by Levesque and Childers. Management of complications of diabetes is discussed in several of the articles. Gibson and Abbas discuss limb salvage; Levesque discusses hypertension management, and Glover and Galvan discuss heart failure. Diabetes education of children by Schreiner and of adults by Keaveny is important so that the patient and family can learn to self-manage their diabetes after discharge. Insulin pumps are not commonly seen in hospitalized

Crit Care Nurs Clin N Am 25 (2013) xi–xii
http://dx.doi.org/10.1016/j.ccell.2013.01.001
0899-5885/13/$ – see front matter © 2013 Published by Elsevier Inc.

ccnursing.theclinics.com

patients and McCrea discusses the basics of insulin pump therapy as well as trouble-shooting and nursing care while the patient is using the pump.

Celia M. Levesque, RN, MSN, NP-C, CNS-BC, BC-ADM, CDE
Department of Endocrine Neoplasia
and Hormonal Disorders
The University of Texas MD Anderson Cancer Center
PO Box 301402-Unit 1461
Houston, TX 77230-1402, USA

E-mail address:
clevesqu@mdanderson.org

Guidelines for Care of the Hospitalized Patient with Hyperglycemia and Diabetes

Kate Crawford, RN, MSN, ANP-C, BC-ADM

KEYWORDS

- Diabetes • Hyperglycemia • Diabetes medications • Insulin • Hypoglycemia

KEY POINTS

- Hyperglycemia and diabetes place hospitalized patients at greater risk for serious complications such as infections, diabetic ketoacidosis, hyperosmolar hyperglycemic state, dehydration, electrolyte imbalances, greater antibiotic use, and lengthened hospitalization.
- Identification and proper treatment of hyperglycemia and diabetes are essential for prevention of significant morbidity and mortality to the patient and to conserve ever-shrinking health care resources.
- It important for the nurse to understand current recommendations for diabetes treatment in the non–critically ill hospitalized patient.

HYPERGLYCEMIA AND DIABETES IN THE HOSPITAL

It is well known that the number of persons with diabetes in the United States is reaching epidemic levels and is expected to grow. In 2011, the Centers for Disease Control and Prevention reported that 8.3% of the US population had diabetes.[1] As the number of persons with diabetes is growing, it is expected that the percentage of hospitalized persons with diabetes will continue to grow. In 2009, diabetes was the second most frequent primary diagnosis noted on hospital discharge in patients aged 18 years and older.[2] The prevalence of diabetes in community hospitals has been reported to range from 32% to 38%.[2] The estimate is dramatically higher, 70% to 80%, in patients with acute coronary syndrome or those undergoing cardiovascular surgery.[3]

Much research has been focused on the best practice for the management of hyperglycemia in specific subgroups of inpatients such as those in perioperative, cardiovascular postsurgical, and intensive care.[4] Numerous studies report reduced rates of infection, length of hospitalization, and mortality with tight glycemic control in these

Disclosure: The author has no relationship with a commercial company that has a direct financial interest in the subject matter or materials discussed in the article or with a company making a competing product.
Department of Endocrine Neoplasia and Hormonal Disorders, The University of Texas MD Anderson Cancer Center, 1515 Holcombe Boulevard, Unit 1461, Houston, TX 77030, USA
E-mail address: kcrawford@mdanderson.org

specific populations. As with critically ill patients, hyperglycemia in non–critically ill hospitalized patients has also been associated with lengthened hospital stay, more infections, and increased mortality.[4] Unfortunately, less data are available for hospitalized patients with hyperglycemia who are not in intensive care. Guidelines for the treatment of inpatient hyperglycemia can be found from numerous expert sources such as the American Diabetes Association (ADA), the American Association of Clinical Endocrinologists (AACE), and the Endocrine Society. In 2009, the ADA and the AACE published a consensus statement on inpatient glycemic control, which will serve as the main reference for this article. This article will discuss the identification of hyperglycemia, assessment of the patient with hyperglycemia, glycemic targets, treatment of hyperglycemia and hypoglycemia, and transition to outpatient care of non–critically ill hospitalized patients.

IDENTIFICATION OF HYPERGLYCEMIA AND DIABETES IN THE HOSPITAL

Hyperglycemia and diabetes are associated with longer hospitalizations, more antibiotic use, more time spent in critical care, and worse overall mortality.[4,5] Unfortunately, for many patients, if diabetes is not the primary diagnosis on admission, the management of hyperglycemia and diabetes is often viewed as less important than the illness that precipitated admission to the hospital. Hyperglycemia in the hospital is not limited to those patients with a known diagnosis of diabetes. In patients without diabetes, transient elevations in glucose can result from numerous factors such as increased catecholamine production, medications such as glucocorticoids, treatments such as parenteral or enteral nutrition, or surgical procedures. In patients being treated for cancer, one study noted worse overall outcomes for those patients with no formal diagnosis of diabetes than for those patients with diagnosed diabetes (P. Shah, MD Anderson Cancer Center, unpublished data, 2009). Because nearly one third of persons with diabetes in the United States are undiagnosed, a significant number of patients may have unrecognized hyperglycemia on hospital admission.[1] Hyperglycemia, regardless of the cause, is an independent predictor of increased morbidity in hospitalized patients.[5] Therefore, to prevent serious complications, it is necessary to identify and treat not only patients with known diabetes but also patients with previously undetected or newly developed hyperglycemia. Hyperglycemia in the hospital is defined as any glucose value greater than140 mg/dL or a hemoglobin A_{1c} value of 5.7% to 6.4%, indicating impaired glucose tolerance, whereas hemoglobin A_{1c} values greater than 6.5% are diagnostic for overt diabetes.[6]

ASSESSING FOR HYPERGLYCEMIA

Patients at high risk for hyperglycemia need to be assessed on admission and throughout their hospitalization for elevated glucose values. For patients with a known diagnosis of diabetes, it is imperative that this diagnosis is noted in the medical record and that glucose monitoring be initiated on admission.[6] Initial assessment of the patient should include at minimum a description of the outpatient medication regimen, level of glycemic control, and frequency of hypoglycemia.

For patients without a history of diabetes or hyperglycemia, glucose monitoring should be initiated in those patients receiving glucocorticoids, enteral or parenteral nutrition, or other medications known to cause hyperglycemia such as octreotide or immunosuppressants.[6]

Patients who are tolerating a diet should have their glucose level monitored before meals and bedtime. Of note, if meals are provided on demand, monitoring should be performed based on the patient's actual meal schedule instead of at fixed intervals.

For patients taking nothing by mouth or receiving continuous enteral or parenteral nutrition, monitoring every 6 hours is sufficient. A hemoglobin A_{1c} level can be checked on admission if not previously measured within the past 3 months, however, a hemoglobin A_{1c} may not indict usual glycemic control in those patients with red blood cell pathologies, those receiving frequent transfusions, or patients with anemia.

GLYCEMIC TARGETS

There are little data to support specific glucose goals outside of critical care.[6] The ADA/AACE consensus statement recommends a preprandial glucose range from 100 to no greater than 140 mg/dL, with random glucose values no greater than 180 mg/dL.[4] They recommend treatment of any glucose value of greater than 180 mg/dL. Glucose values less than 70 mg/dL represent hypoglycemia and should be avoided. In stable patients with previously well-controlled diabetes, lower glucose targets may be appropriate. Less stringent targets are appropriate in patients at high risk for hypoglycemia such as those with hepatic or renal dysfunction, the elderly, patients with altered mental status, or patients for whom tight glycemic control is not clinically beneficial such as those in palliative care.

TREATMENT OF HYPERGLYCEMIA

The ADA/AACE consensus statement recommends treatment of any glucose level greater than 180 mg/dL.[4] The preferred regimen for the treatment of hyperglycemia is with scheduled subcutaneous injections of insulin, which includes 3 components: basal, bolus, and correctional.[6] Basal insulin is provided to control glucose elevations from hepatic glucose output between meals and during sleep. Basal insulin is long-acting and is administered only once or twice daily. Because patients with type 1 diabetes are absolutely insulin deficient, it is critical that they receive basal insulin daily, regardless of nutritional status, to prevent diabetic ketoacidosis. Bolus insulin is provided to control glucose elevations that result from food intake. Bolus insulin is typically rapid or short-acting and is administered before meals only. It is important to administer bolus insulin based on the actual timing of the patient's meal instead of on standardized or predetermined hospital administration times. Correctional insulin is a dose of rapid or short-acting insulin, usually administered with a bolus dose to correct for high glucose before a meal. Correctional doses of insulin without regard to meals or at bedtime should be avoided to prevent hypoglycemia. Insulin regimens should be reassessed if glucose values are less than 100, as the patient is at risk for hypoglycemia.[4] Insulin regimens need to be adjusted if glucose values decrease to less than 70 mg/dL.[4] Patients who use continuous subcutaneous infusions of insulin via insulin pumps can continue to manage their diabetes while in the hospital only if they are willing and cognitively capable of independently managing the insulin pump. Nursing staff must document patient-administered basal and bolus insulin doses administered via the insulin pump. Infusion sites should be changed at a minimum every 72 hours.

"Sliding scale" insulin should not be used for hyperglycemia lasting longer than 24 hours.[7] If patients experience persistent elevations in glucose, a physiologic insulin program using basal, bolus, and correction insulin should be instituted.[8] Sliding scale protocols do not deliver insulin in a physiologic fashion, resulting in wide glucose variability. In addition, sliding scale insulin places the patient at greater risk for hypoglycemia because it is usually administered without regard to meals.[7] Patients with type 1 diabetes require scheduled injections of basal insulin, despite nutritional status, and therefore should never be prescribed sliding scale insulin alone as treatment of their diabetes. The use of noninsulin treatments for hyperglycemia in the hospital is discouraged.[4] Hospitalized patients can have rapidly deteriorating hepatic and renal function, widely variable nutrition intake, and frequent medication changes. They often undergo unscheduled testing with contrast media that is contraindicated for use with some oral diabetes medications. **Table 1** provides a list of noninsulin diabetes medications and their indications for use in hospitalized patients. For a detailed discussion of insulin and oral regimens, please refer to the articles by Levesque and Martin in this issue.

TREATMENT OF HYPOGLYCEMIA

Hypoglycemia is the central limiting factor in the treatment of hyperglycemia and is a critical component of hyperglycemia management.[6] Hypoglycemia is defined as a glucose value of less than 70 mg/dL, with severe hypoglycemia defined as a glucose

Table 1 Noninsulin diabetes medications and indications for use in hospitalized patients	
Medication Names, Generic (Brand)	**Use in Hospital**
Oral Diabetes Medications	
Sulfonylureas: Glimepiride (Amaryl) Glipizide (Glucotrol, Glucotrol XL) Glyburide (Diabeta, Glynase PresTab, Micronase)	Discontinue: high risk for hypoglycemia due to unpredictable PO intake, fasting, elevated creatinine
Meglitinides: Nateglinide (Starlix) Repaglinide (Prandin)	Discontinue: high risk for hypoglycemia because of unpredictable oral intake or fasting
Thiazolidinediones: Pioglitazone (Actos) Rosiglitizone (Avandia)	Can continue in stable patients because they do not cause hypoglycemia. Do not initiate in patients with congestive heart failure or edema
Biguanides: Metformin (Glucophage, Glucophage XR, Fortamet, Riomet)	Hold: for creatinine >1.4 mg/dL women, >1.5 mg/dL in men. Hold after contrast until renal function is verified. Do not initiate in patient with nausea, vomiting, or diarrhea
α-Glucosidase inhibitors: Acarbose (Precose) Miglitol (Glyset)	Discontinue: high risk for hypoglycemia because of unpredictable oral intake, fasting Do not initiate in patient with nausea, vomiting, or diarrhea
Dipeptidyl peptidase-4 inhibitors: Sitagliptin phosphate (Januvia) Saxagliptin (Onglyza), Linagliptin (Tradjenta)	Do not cause hypoglycemia; OK for stable patients or those ready for discharge
Noninsulin Injectable Diabetes Medications	
Incretin mimetics: Exenatide (Byetta) Exenatide extended release (Bydureon) Liraglutide (Victoza)	Do not produce hypoglycemia Caution in gastrointestinal/surgical patients; cause delayed gastric emptying and can cause nausea
Amylin agonists: Pramlintide (Symlin)	Given immediately before meals with rapid-acting insulin; would not be given unless the patient is eating a meal

value of less than 40 mg/dL.[6] Hospitalized patients are at high risk for hypoglycemia because of rapidly changing clinical circumstances such as changes in nutrition status, reduction in glucocorticoids, reduction in dextrose content in intravenous fluids, cessation of total parenteral nutrition or tube feeding, prolonged use of sliding scale insulin therapy, sulfonylurea use, and improper administration of insulin.[6,9] Patients at greatest risk for hypoglycemia include the elderly; the undernourished; those with a history of severe hypoglycemia; patients with hepatic, renal, or cardiac failure; and patients with sepsis. Hypoglycemia can result in serious injury to the patient if not corrected. Standardized hypoglycemia protocols should be implemented for all patients receiving treatment of hyperglycemia.[4] For patients who are alert and able to swallow, 15 g of oral glucose is the preferred treatment.[6] The use of intravenous dextrose 50% should be limited to those patients who are unable to take carbohydrates by mouth. Glucagon can be administered intramuscularly or subcutaneously to revive an unconscious patient in whom intravenous access cannot be established. In patients receiving insulin therapy, care needs to be paid to any change in oral status; the development of nausea, vomiting, or sepsis; and avoidance of nonphysiologic insulin administration to avoid hypoglycemia.

TRANSITION TO OUTPATIENT CARE

Transition from acute care to home can be a stressful time for patients and caregivers. Patients with hyperglycemia have several skills they must master, usually in a short duration of time. This necessitates the need to begin discharge planning and education either on admission or as soon as hyperglycemia is detected to facilitate a smooth transition from hospital to home. At a minimum, patients with hyperglycemia need education on the following areas before discharge[6]:

- Understanding of the diagnosis of diabetes/hyperglycemia, glucose monitoring, and home glucose goals
- Signs, symptoms, and treatment of hypoglycemia
- Signs, symptoms, and treatment of hyperglycemia
- Diet recommendations
- Medication instructions
- Sick day management
- Insulin injection and needle disposal instruction
- Plan for follow up after discharge

Providers must ensure the patient has the appropriate supplies for discharge, including medications, syringes or needles, lancets, test strips, and a glucometer. A certified diabetes educator is an invaluable resource for educating patients and families and should be utilized if available.

SUMMARY

Although there are limited randomized trials supporting a single approach to the management of inpatient hyperglycemia, the ADA/AACE consensus statement provides guidelines. Clinicians need to conduct a thorough admission assessment to screen for diabetes and should be vigilant for hyperglycemia that develops during hospitalization. Treatment of hyperglycemia should focus on physiologic insulin replacement using a basal/bolus/correction regimen rather than sliding scale coverage. Glucose values should be controlled, minimizing acute complications such as hypoglycemia, infections, and increased length of stay.

REFERENCES

1. Centers for Disease Control and Prevention. 2011 National Diabetes Fact Sheet. 2011. Available at: http://www.dcd.gov/diabetes/pubs/estimates11htm. Accessed August 20, 2012.
2. Centers for Disease Control and Prevention. Distribution of first-listed diagnoses among hospital discharges with diabetes as any listed diagnosis, adults aged 18 years and older, United States. 2009. Available at: http://www.cdc.gov/diabetes/statistics/hosp/adulttable1.htm. Accessed August 20, 2012.
3. Smiley D, Umpierrez GE. Management of hyperglycemia in the hospitalized patient. Ann N Y Acad Sci 2010;1212:1–11. http://dx.doi.org/10.1111/j.1749-6632.2010.05805.
4. Moghissi E, Korytkowsi M, DiNardo M, et al. American Association of Clinical Endocrinologists and American Diabetes Association consensus statement on inpatient glycemic control. Diabetes Care 2009;32:1119–31.
5. Lieva RR, Inzucchi SE. Hospital management of hyperglycemia. Curr Opin Endocrinol Diabetes Obes 2011;18:110–8. http://dx.doi.org/10.1097/MED.0b013e3283447a6d.
6. American Diabetes Association. Standards of medical care in diabetes: 2012. Diabetes Care 2012;35(Suppl 1):S11–63.
7. Kitabchi AE, Nyenue E. Sliding scale insulin: more evidence needed before the final exit? Diabetes Care 2007;30:2409–10.
8. Umpierrez GE, Smiley D, Jacobs S, et al. Randomized study of basal-bolus insulin therapy in the inpatient management of patients with type 2 diabetes undergoing general surgery (RABBIT 2 surgery). Diabetes Care 2011;34:256–61.
9. Umpierrez GE, Palacio A, Smiley D. Sliding scale insulin use: myth or insanity? Am J Med 2007;120:563–7.

Management of Hyperglycemia in the Intensive Care Unit
When Glucose Reaches Critical Levels

Veronica Brady, MSN, FNP-BC, BC-ADM, CDE

KEYWORDS

- Blood glucose • Hyperglycemia • Insulin • Intensive care unit

KEY POINTS

- Hyperglycemia among hospitalized critically ill patients is an independent predictor of poorer outcomes.
- Appropriate treatment of hyperglycemia among these patients is associated with reduced mortality and morbidity.
- The goal of treatment of hyperglycemia in the critically ill patient is to achieve glycemic control without causing undo hypoglycemia.

INTRODUCTION

Hyperglycemia among hospitalized patients is not a new phenomenon. Over the last several decades much attention has been given to the risks, benefits, and recommendations for the management of hyperglycemia among hospitalized patients. Inpatient hyperglycemia is often associated with a diagnosis of diabetes. According to the American Diabetes Association there are currently 25.8 million persons in the United States (8.3% of the population) living with a diagnosis of diabetes.[1] Although the exact number of patients that experience hyperglycemia during the course of admission is unknown, according to the Centers for Disease Control and Prevention 5.5 million hospital discharges in 2009 listed diabetes among the diagnosis.[2] It was also estimated that 22% of all patient days were incurred by patients with diabetes.[3] As stated by Smiley and Umpierrez,[4] the prevalence of hyperglycemia among patients in community hospitals has ranged from 32% to 38% and from approximately 70% to 80% in patients with acute coronary syndrome and cardiac surgery, respectively.

Disclosure: The author has no relationship with a commercial company that has a direct financial interest in the subject matter or materials discussed in the article or with a company making a competing product.
Department of Endocrine Neoplasia and Hormonal Disorders, The University of Texas MD Anderson Cancer Center, PO Box 301402-Unit 1461, Houston, TX 77030-1402, USA
E-mail address: vbrady@mdanderson.org

Hyperglycemia in the hospitalized patient is an independent predictor of poorer outcomes,[5] and was also thought to be an indicator of severity of illness.[6] Critically ill patients who develop hyperglycemia have been shown to be at increased risk for hospital complications; increased mortality; longer lengths of stay (resulting in high hospital cost); and increased septicemia.[4] Although studies examining the risks and benefits of tight glycemic control along with debates about how tight is too tight to control glucose in the critical care setting continues, the evidence does suggest that management of hyperglycemia improves patient outcomes. Although research persists it behooves those practicing in the intensive care setting to recognize that hyperglycemia is an issue, know who is at risk, and use best practices for glucose management.

HYPERGLYCEMIA DEFINED

Hyperglycemia in the hospitalized patient is not only seen among patients with diabetes. Stress hyperglycemia, steroid-induced hyperglycemia, stress diabetes, and "transient" hospital-related hyperglycemia are also often seen. At a glance it is difficult to ascertain whether a patient is hyperglycemic as a result from having diabetes and antidiabetic medications being withheld or administered incorrectly, or if the patient is experiencing hyperglycemia caused by stress. Regardless of the reason for the glucose elevation it is imperative that a standardized definition be used to identify the phenomenon.

Traditionally, hyperglycemia was defined as random glucose readings of greater than 200 mg/dL, and treatment was not initiated until the threshold for glycemic-related complications was reached. At the time of the Leuven study hyperglycemia was defined as blood glucose concentrations greater than 110 mg/dL (6.1 mmol/L) and it was estimated that 80% to 90% of patients in the intensive care unit (ICU) experienced hyperglycemia.[7] Subsequently, the Normoglycemia in Intensive Care Evaluation-Survival Using Glucose Algorithm Regulation trial reported that blood glucose targets of 81 to 108 mg/dL resulted in higher mortality and a target of l80 mg/dL resulted in lower mortality.[8] Following this study the American Association of Clinical Endocrinologists and American Diabetes Association produced a consensus statement that defined hyperglycemia as blood glucose greater than 140 mg/dL (>7.8 mmol/L).[3,8] American Diabetes Association 2012 Guidelines offer clear definitions of diabetes, prediabetes, glucose targets, and suggestions of targets for glycemic control among patients with critical illness.[9] **Table 1** provides definitions of diabetes, hyperglycemia, and hypoglycemia, and glycemic targets.

Table 1
Definitions and glycemic targets (American Diabetes Association 2012 Guidelines)

Diagnosis	Definition Results (mg/dL)	Glycemic Targets
Diabetes	Fasting glucose ≥126 Random glucose ≥200 A_{1c} >6.5%–7%	Preprandial glucose 70–130 Peak postprandial <180 A_{1c} <7%
Inpatient hyperglycemia	Blood glucose >140	Blood glucose 140–180 (110–140 in surgical patients)
Persistent hyperglycemia	Requiring treatment 180	
Classic hyperglycemia (hyperglycemic crisis)	Blood glucose ≥200	
Hypoglycemia	Blood glucose <70	
Severe hypoglycemia	Blood glucose ≤40	

CAUSES OF HYPERGLYCEMIA AMONG CRITICALLY ILL PATIENTS

Hyperglycemia in the critically ill patient occurs as a result of various factors.[10] Among patients with known history of diabetes the elevation in glucose may be related to lack of administration of antidiabetic medications, particularly for those on oral agents. For patients who are insulin dependent, glucose elevations may occur as a result of withholding usual insulin doses or use of sliding scale insulin. In patients without previous diagnosis of diabetes glucose elevations may be an indicator of previously undiagnosed diabetes. The most reliable method for ascertaining the presence of underlying diabetes is by obtaining a hemoglobin A_{1c}. According to the American Diabetes Association a diagnosis of diabetes can be made with A_{1c} of greater than or equal to 6.5%. A_{1c} levels and the corresponding glucose are listed in **Table 2**.

In those patients lacking a diagnosis of diabetes, whether diagnosed or underlying, hyperglycemia can result from increased adrenaline, cortisol, catecholamines, growth hormone, glucagon, glycogenolysis, gluconeogenesis, and insulin resistance.[10] **Table 3** provides the causes of hyperglycemia and hypoglycemia in the critically ill patient. Before the Leuven study in 2001 these elevations in glucose had been considered to be a normal, adaptive response, which was of benefit to the patient in that it prevented hypoglycemia.

MANAGEMENT OF HYPERGLYCEMIA IN CRITICALLY ILL PATIENTS

Regardless of the term used to define it or the cause, hyperglycemia in the critically ill patient must be addressed. Although oral agents can be used to assist in the management of hyperglycemia in hospital, their use is not recommended for the critically ill patient. The benefits of insulin therapy compared with oral agents are outlined in **Table 4**. Insulin therapy is the drug of choice among this population. Insulin is known to decrease hepatic glucose production and increase glucose "disposal"; it is effective and has unlimited efficacy.[11] However, insulin must be used with caution. According to diabetes management guidelines insulin should not be initiated unless the patient displays persistent hyperglycemia (blood glucose >180 mg/dL). Insulin administered subcutaneously or by insulin drip are the two methods that can be used. There are a variety of insulins available for inpatient use (**Table 5**). However, regular insulin should be used for intravenous formulations. If patients are not taking anything by mouth, regular insulin can be administered subcutaneously every 6 hours. For patients with oral intake, any of the analog insulins at the time of the meal would likely be beneficial.

Table 2		
Blood glucose and corresponding hemoglobin A_{1c}		
	Mean Plasma Blood Glucose	
Hemoglobin A_{1c} %	**mg/dL**	**mmol/L**
6	126	7
7	154	8.6
8	183	10.2
9	212	11.8
10	240	13.4
11	269	14.9
12	298	16.5

Data from American Diabetes Association. Standards of medical care in diabetes: 2012. Diabetes Care 2012;35:S11–63.

Table 3 Causes of hyperglycemia and hypoglycemia in the critically ill patient	
Hyperglycemia	**Hypoglycemia**
Total parenteral nutrition	Infection/sepsis
Glucocorticosteroids	Hepatic failure
Exogenous catecholamines	Renal failure
Insulin resistance	Surgery
Intravenous dextrose	Insulin-secreting tumors
Release of stress hormones (epinephrine and cortisol)	Lack of nutritional intake (NPO status)/cachexia
Gluconeogenesis (liver)	
Lipolysis (fat cells)	

Data from Hassall S, Butler-Williams C. Blood glucose monitoring in critically ill patients. Br J Neurosci Nurs 2010;6:342–4; and Kavanagh BP, McCowen KC. Glycemia control in the ICU. N Engl J Med 2010;363:2540–6.

Subcutaneous insulin and insulin by drip protocol require that patients undergo frequent blood glucose monitoring. In the critical care setting this is often done by obtaining a blood specimen from an arterial (central) line. These results are often preferred in that it avoids the patient having a finger stick and the specimen can be obtained quickly. The downside to arterial line blood draws is that often these patients are receiving intravenous fluids that contain dextrose or various other additives that can affect the results of the glucose reading if the line is not flushed properly before drawing the specimen. By that same token capillary (finger stick) blood glucose readings can also be unreliable because of user error or patients' clinical condition. Patient conditions that affect glucose readings are reviewed in **Table 6**. Caution should be used when interpreting point-of-care glucose readings in patients with edema, poor peripheral perfusion, and in cases where an adequate sample was not obtained.[12]

Whether patients have known history of diabetes, are found to have underlying diabetes during critical illness, or if they are experiencing stress-induced hyperglycemia, they all require appropriate glucose management. Current recommendations are to initiate insulin therapy when glucose reaches 180 mg/dL and titrate insulin to maintain glucose between 140 and 180 mg/dL. Insulin therapy should be discontinued when glucose reaches target levels.

Patients with a known history of diabetes may benefit from higher blood glucose levels than their nondiabetic counterparts. Hyperglycemia among this patient population has not been shown to result in a worse prognosis.[13]

Table 4 Comparison of insulin with oral hypoglycemics	
Insulin	**Oral Hypoglycemics**
No interactions	Not effective in severe hyperglycemia
Quick onset and clearance	Medical interactions-study medicines, IV contrast, heart failure
No dose limitations	Delayed onset
Rare side effects	Prolonged clearance in renal insufficiency
	Side effects-N/V/D, edema

Table 5				

Types of insulin and duration of action				
Insulin Type	**Product**	**Onset**	**Peak**	**Duration**
Rapid-Acting				
Aspart	Novolog	10–30 min	30 min to 3 h	3–5 h
Glulisine	Apidra			
Lispro	Humalog			
Short–Acting				
Regular	HumulinR	30–60 min	2–5 h	Up to 12 h
	Novolin R			
Intermediate-Acting				
NPH	Humulin N	90 min to 4 h	4–12 h	Up to 24 h*
	Humulin R			
Long-Acting				
Detemir	Levemir	45 min to 4 h	Minimal peak	Up to 24 h*
Glargine	Lantus			
Combination Insulin				
	70/30, 75/25, 50/50	10–15 min	10–15 h	14–18 h

* Indicates that the duration of action may be more or less than 24 hours.

GLYCEMIC CONTROL IN THE CRITICALLY ILL PATIENT
Risks of Treatment

The primary risk associated with glycemic management in any patient population is that of hypoglycemia. The same is true of the critically ill patient. Hypoglycemia among these patients increases the risk of death. This risk is greater among patients that experience spontaneous hypoglycemia than those being treated with insulin therapy. According to Gunst and Van den Berghe,[14] this hypoglycemia may be indicative of the severity of illness. Often in the critically ill patient it is difficult to detect the presence of hypoglycemia. Studies have reported that up to 4 years after an inpatient hypoglycemic event patients have been shown to have impaired social functioning and quality of life.[13] Although hypoglycemia puts patients at increased risk for death, wide fluctuations in glucose (glycemic variability) has also been shown to be an independent risk factor for ICU and hospital mortality.[15]

Hypoglycemia signs and symptoms increase in severity as the glucose decreases: at 70 mg/dL, counterregulatory hormones are released; at 60 mg/dL, glucagon is

Table 6	

Conditions impacting blood glucose readings	
False Elevations	**False Depressions**
Hypoxia	Hematocrit >55%
Hyperlipidemia	Intravenous infusion of ascorbic acid
Anemia/hematocrit <35%	Severe dehydration
Dialysis	Shock (peripheral circulatory failure)
Jaundice (bilirubin >0.43 mmol/L)	

Data from Hassall S, Butler-Williams C. Blood glucose monitoring in critically ill patients. Br J Neurosci Nurs 2010;6:342–4; and Flower O, Finfer S. Glucose control in critically ill patients. Intern Med J 2012;42:4–6.

Table 7
Risk/benefit from glycemic control (blood glucose 80–100 mg/dL)

Critical Care Setting	Risk	Benefit
Cardiac		↓ Infection ↓ Mortality
Medical	Six fold ↑ hypoglycemia	↓ Morbidity ↓ Mortality
Surgical		↓ Morbidity ↓ Mortality

released; at 50 mg/dL adrenergic symptoms from epinephrine and norepinephrine, diaphoresis, tremor, palpitations, and tachycardia occur; at 20 to 40 mg/dL, neuroglycopenic symptoms, impaired consciousness, and seizures can occur; and at 10 mg/dL permanent blindness and paralysis may occur.

Benefits of Treatment

Although risk of hypoglycemia is real, multiple studies have shown that appropriate management of hyperglycemia during the time of critical illness is beneficial in certain patient populations (**Table 7**). The use of insulin therapy has been reported to reverse lipolysis, vasoconstriction, platelet aggregation, overproduction of free fatty acids, and inflammation.[4]

NOVEL APPROACHES TO GLUCOSE MANAGEMENT

Management of hyperglycemia in the ICU requires a team that is skilled in the use of insulin therapy.[16,17] Although the use of intravenous insulin is the usual method used to manage hyperglycemia in the critical care setting, the risk of hypoglycemia and issues with the reliability of the test results often makes this task challenging. Over the past several years researchers have implemented the use of the Glucommander and continuous glucose infusion to achieve tighter glycemic control without adverse effects and potentially decrease the amount of nursing time associated with managing patients on insulin drips. When compared with standard insulin protocols, use of the Glucommander (Davidson, Atlanta, GA) (computerized decision support) has been associated with less glycemic variability, decreased time required to achieve glucose targets, and tighter glycemic control with higher incidences of hypoglycemia.[5] The closed loop system (continuous glucose infusion) has been shown to lower the risk of poor outcomes among patients admitted to the ICU after open heart surgery. Continuous glucose monitoring systems have also been and are currently being studied to see if they provide accurate glucose readings and to determine if their use is tolerated in the critically ill patient.

SUMMARY

How to best manage hyperglycemia in the critically ill patient remains an area that requires further investigation. The debate continues about how tight glucose control should be for patients to experience maximum benefit without suffering from hypoglycemia. What is known, however, is that management of hyperglycemia without causing undo hypoglycemia results in improved patient outcomes, intravenous insulin administration is usually the most effective, treatment should begin as soon as possible, and hyperglycemia in the critically ill patient should not be tolerated.

REFERENCES

1. American Diabetes Association. Diabetes statistics. Available at: http://www. diabetes.org/diabetes-basics/diabetes-statistics/. Accessed September 8, 2012.
2. Centers for Disease Control and Prevention. National diabetes fact sheet. 2011. Available at: http://www.cdc.gov/diabetes/pubs/pdf/ndfs_2011.pdf. Accessed September 8, 2012.
3. Moghissi E, Korytkowski M, DiNardo M, et al. American Association of Clinical Endocrinologists and American Diabetes Association consensus statement on inpatient glycemic control. Diabetes Care 2009;32:1119–31. http://dx.doi.org/10.2337/dc09-9029.
4. Smiley D, Umpierrez G. Management of hyperglycemia in the hospitalized patients. Ann N Y Acad Sci 2010;12:1–11. http://dx.doi.org/10.1111/j.1749-6632.2010.05805.
5. Lleva R, Inzucchi SE. Hospital management of hyperglycemia. Curr Opin Endocrinol Diabetes Obes 2011;18:110–8. http://dx.doi.org/10.1097/MED.0b013e3283447a6d.
6. Preiser JC, Devos P, Chiolero R. Which factors influence glycemic control in the intensive care unit? Curr Opin Clin Nutr Metab Care 2010;13:205–10. http://dx.doi.org/10.1097/MC).0b013e328335720b.
7. Egi M, Finfer S, Bellomo R. Glycemic control in the ICU. Chest 2011;140:212–20. http://dx.doi.org/10.1378/chest.10-1478.
8. The NICE-SUGAR Study Investigators. Intensive versus conventional glucose control in critically ill patients. N Engl J Med 2009;360:1283–97. http://dx.doi.org/10.1056/NEJMoa810625.
9. American Diabetes Association. Standards of medical care in diabetes: 2012. Diabetes Care 2012;35:S11–63.
10. Stapleton RD, Heyland DK. Glycemic control and intensive insulin therapy in critical illness. 2011. Available at: www.uptodate.com. Accessed May 21, 2012.
11. Inzucchi SE, Bergenstal RM, Buse JB, et al. Management of hyperglycemia in type 2 diabetes: a patient-centered approach. Position statement of the American Diabetes Association (ADA) and the European Association for the Study of Diabetes (EASD). Diabetes Care 2012;35:1364–79. http://dx.doi.org/10.1007/s00125-012-2534-0.
12. Hassall S, Butler-Williams C. Blood glucose monitoring in critically ill patients. Br J Neurosci Nurs 2010;6:342–4.
13. Kavanagh BP, McCowen KC. Glycemia control in the ICU. N Engl J Med 2010;363:2540–6. http://dx.doi.org/10.1056/NEJMcp100115.
14. Gunst J, Van den Berghe G. Blood glucose control in the intensive care unit: benefits and risk. Semin Dial 2010;23:157–62. http://dx.doi.org/10.1111/j.1525-139X.2010.00702.x.
15. Al-Dorzi HM, Tamim HA, Arabi YM. Glycaemic fluctuation predicts mortality in critically ill patients. Anaesth Intensive Care 2010;38:695–702.
16. Fahy BG, Sheeny AM, Coursin DB. Glucose control in the intensive care unit. Crit Care Med 2009;37:1769–76. http://dx.doi.org/10.1097/CCM.0b013e3181a19ceb.
17. Flower O, Finfer S. Glucose control in critically ill patients. Intern Med J 2012;42:4–6. http://dx.doi.org/10.1111/j.1445-5994.2011.02631.x.

Intravenous Insulin Infusions
What Nurses Need to Know

Ashley Martin, MSN, RN, ANP-BC

KEYWORDS

- Intravenous insulin infusion • Acute care • Insulin drip • Glucose control
- Insulin protocol • Computer-based system

KEY POINTS

- Insulin drip can help achieve blood glucose targets and minimize hypoglycemia in intensive care patients.
- Multiple drip protocols and methods for delivering the insulin exist.
- Nurses play a vital role in helping to identify patients in need of intravenous insulin, initiating the drip, educating the patient and family, calculating rates or using computerized rate calculations, and managing transition to subcutaneous insulin.

INTRODUCTION

Glucose control in the acute setting has long been a debate among leaders in the fields of diabetes and acute care. In 2001, Van Den Berghe and colleagues[1] introduced the benefit of tight glucose control in the critical care setting with findings of approximately 50% reduced mortality when glucose was maintained no higher than 110 mg/dL. Following this study, there was evidence that tight glucose control with parameters up to 110 mg/dL versus 180 mg/dL led to an increased rate of hypoglycemia and mortality.[2–5] The latest consensus by the American Association of Clinical Endocrinologists and the American Diabetes Association (ADA) for glucose control in the critical care setting is to initiate insulin therapy for glucose levels higher than 180 mg/dL and to maintain the blood glucose at 140 to 180 mg/dL.[6] The ADA added that a goal of 110 to 140 mg/dL may be recommended in select patients as long as it can be maintained without increased risk of hypoglycemia.[7] Providers work to maintain euglycemia in critically ill patients with tight control and low rates of hypoglycemia; however, this has proved difficult.

Patients in the intensive care unit (ICU) have many variables that interfere with glucose control including infection, lack of consistent nutrition and food by mouth,

Disclosures: The author has no affiliations to disclose.
Department of Endocrine Neoplasia and Hormonal Disorders, M.D. Anderson Cancer Center, 1400 Pressler Street, Unit 1461, Houston, TX 77030, USA
E-mail address: akmartin@mdanderson.org

renal and liver damage, administration of steroids, and stress, leading to increased endogenous steroid production. Subcutaneous insulin requires longer intervals of glucose testing and is difficult to adjust to rapidly changing situations. Intravenous insulin infusions are frequently preferred in the critical care setting to control glucose, because they can be titrated for changing insulin requirements and can be cleared from the system rapidly. Nurses managing intravenous insulin infusions in the critical care setting rely on established algorithms to assist in effective titration of infusion rates. Currently, there are numerous protocols in use that promise accurate glycemic control and are capable of maintaining levels within a tight range with low rates of hypoglycemia. This article reviews the basics of insulin infusions, a small selection of frequently used protocols, and the role of nursing in glucose control in the acute care setting.

INSULIN INFUSION BASICS
Indication

Continuous intravenous insulin is the recommended treatment of hyperglycemia in the critical care setting.[7] This includes the management of known diabetic patients, or nondiabetic patients with hyperglycemia. It has been proven safe and effective to use insulin drips in this setting with a low risk of hypoglycemia, regardless of which algorithm is used. Insulin infusions are essential in the quick resolution of conditions such as diabetic ketoacidosis and hyperosmolar nonketotic state.[8] Cardiac and vascular conditions have also shown significant benefit with stable glucose control on insulin infusions and should be considered in all such cases.[9,10] These conditions include myocardial infarction, cardiogenic shock, stroke, and cardiac surgeries and procedures. Other indications for insulin infusion include sepsis, parenteral nutrition, nothing by mouth in diabetic patients, and initiation of steroids; additionally, it should be used for diabetic women in labor and during delivery.[11]

Initiation of Infusion

Insulin infusions are comprised of regular insulin 100 units mixed in 100 mL of normal saline. Each protocol differs on whether an initial bolus dose of insulin is indicated when the infusion is started. There is also a difference in opinion on whether simultaneous glucose should be infused while intravenous insulin is running. In 2008, 64% of published insulin protocols recommended continuous glucose infusions or enteral feeding with administration of intravenous insulin.[12] Once the insulin infusion is initiated, it is important to establish a clear and consistent way to document all glucose readings and dose adjustments. If a paper-based protocol is used, nurses should make all calculations in a quiet area to reduce distractions and errors. Regardless of the protocol used, insulin infusions require frequent glucose testing, and all readings must be performed in a timely manner.

Transitioning to Subcutaneous Insulin

One mistake made frequently in practice is the discontinuation of intravenous insulin without a well-devised plan for subcutaneous insulin administration. The result of transitioning a patient from continuous intravenous insulin to sliding scale insulin alone is severe hyperglycemia. A recommended calculation to use is to determine the total insulin delivered intravenously over the last 8 hours and multiply by 3. This is the approximate current 24-hours intravenous insulin requirement. Calculate 40% of this as the basal insulin dose and 40% divided equally into 3 for the prandial doses. The best time to initiate subcutaneous insulin is before a meal. Doses must be given before insulin infusion discontinued. If the patient is not eating, it is recommended to continue managing with intravenous insulin.

Computerized Versus Manual Algorithms

The calculation of insulin adjustments to meet the needs of individual patients requires a combination of inclusiveness that takes many variables into account and simplicity of use that reduces errors when implemented. The current algorithms can be divided into 2 categories, computer-based systems and paper-based protocols (PBPs). PBPs consist of multiple protocols created and tested by nurses and physicians at various institutions. They are presented as written instructions to the nurse directing adjustments and monitoring intervals based on past and current glucose values. PBP examples include the Portland Protocol and the Yale University protocol.[13] Computer-based systems are systems created to calculate insulin dose adjustments based on mathematical control theory.[13] Each program is designed differently, with the capability to take multiple variables into account to recommend dose changes and glucose testing frequency. There are multiple programs available; 2 examples include the Glucommander[11,14] and the Glucostabilizer.[15]

PBPs have been useful for many years, providing a visual and tangible method for dosage calculations. They are dependent on nurse-controlled management and accuracy, which can lead to errors. With increasing workload on nursing staff, it is difficult to integrate extra variables into a PBP, or it may be too cumbersome to follow and possibly increase error rate. They are best used in patients who are not eating anything by mouth, as many do not incorporate meal boluses. Well-established PBPs have been improved and updated to remain competitive with computer-based systems. Overall, many PBPs will effectively lower blood glucose to the targeted range[13]; however, they have a higher rate of hypoglycemia compared with computer-based systems.[16–18]

Like the PBP, each computer-based system uses different methods and calculations for dose adjustments, some more aggressive than others. They are accessed by the nurse through handheld computers or a desktop computer or laptop computer. Some are installed programs, and others are Web-based through the secure institution intranet. Many have the capability to report glucose values and other data in graphs to assess trends. This is helpful information to the nurses caring for the patients and the providers. An increase in nursing compliance has been found with computer-based systems compared with PBPs; however, there are more, on average, glucose measurements taken over the course of the day.[18]

Protocols

When choosing an algorithm to use in a particular setting, one must look at all the attributes of paper-based versus computer-based systems as well as all the features of each individual algorithm before selecting. The following sections contain a small sampling of insulin infusion protocols widely used today.

Portland protocol

The Portland protocol is a product of the Portland Diabetes Project based out of the Providence Heart and Diabetes Institute. It was first used in 1992 and has been continuously updated over the years. Extensive data were published on patient outcomes in the surgical ICU following cardiac surgery from 1987 to 2005 as the protocol evolved.[19] The target glucose range was lowered and tightened to a range of 70 to 110 mg/dL in 2005. Of those treated, 91% of patients reached range within the first 3 hours of initiating protocol, and the rate of hypoglycemia was 1.5%.[20] The average blood glucose of all patients treated on the protocol at the host hospital in 2005 was 121 mg/dL.[19] Insulin dosing is based on the glucose level and rate of change. It does not account for insulin sensitivity.[20] The Web site offers several versions of the protocol including different target rages for ICU use and floor use.

Yale insulin infusion protocol
The Yale protocol was published in a study by Goldberg and colleagues[21] in 2004. The target glucose range was identified as 100 to 139 mg/dL. The documented mean time to achieve the target range was 10.1 hours. Sixty-six percent of glucose readings in the study reached a clinically desirable range of 80 to 139 mg/dL. Twenty readings out of 5808 (0.3%) were below 60 mg/dL.[21] The infusion is started with a bolus dose of insulin, which does not occur in the Portland protocol. Insulin dose changes are calculated based on glucose reading and rate of change.[13]

Glucommander system
Glucommander was first established in a hospital in Atlanta, Georgia on 1984 and was adjusted and updated until the first publication of data in 2005.[11] At that time, the target range changed over the years, but the majority of the time, it was 80 to 120 mg/dL. The protocol has been used mostly on medical/surgical floors, but it has also been used in emergency rooms, operating rooms, and delivery suites. Of all glucose readings captured during the 120,683 hours of infusion, only 0.6% dropped below 50 mg/dL. Time to reaching mean glucose of less than 150 mg/dL was 3 hours.[11] Glucommander is now owned by Glytec, and it has evolved significantly over the years since the initial publication. It currently operates as a Web-based system that produces data reports, assists with transition to subcutaneous insulin, and offers a meal bolus feature.

Glucostabilizer system
The Glucostabilizer system was first published on 2007 by Junega and colleagues.[15] The system was created to account for patient-specific insulin sensitivity when advising insulin adjustments. Insulin sensitivity and target range are programmable at the time of system initiation. Doses and testing intervals are based on glucose readings and rate of change. The system offers bolus doses for meals based on a set insulin-to-carbohydrate ratio. The setting of use includes the ICU, progressive care units, and medical/surgical floors. Initial published data in 2007 were in an ICU with a target range of 80 to 110 mg/dL. Sixty-one percent of glucose readings fell in the target range, with a hypoglycemia rate, defined as less than 50 mg/dL, of 0.4%. Average blood glucose was 106.5 mg/dL.[15]

Nursing Considerations
Technologic advances have changed the way we practice in the medical field over the last several decades. Most advances have proved useful in increasing accuracy, minimizing work load, and improving communication. There is not currently a commercially available system that will integrate a continuous glucose monitor with a computer-based insulin delivery system that will make dose adjustments without significant nurse involvement. Although this type of system may be available soon, the nurse continues to play a key role in the management of hyperglycemia in the acute care setting. Nurses are responsible for helping to identify patients in need of intravenous insulin, initiating drips, education of patient and families, manually calculating rates or using computerized rate calculations, and managing transition to subcutaneous insulin. Whether a PBP or a computer-based system is adopted to manage glucose, it is important for the nurse to become familiarized with the overall process. It is a nurse's responsibility to work alongside providers to reduce the

mortality rate in the acute care setting. Using insulin infusions accurately and selecting the protocol that matches best with each institution are well-established ways to achieve this goal.

REFERENCES

1. Van den Berghe G, Wouters P, Weekers F, et al. Intensive insulin therapy in critically ill patients. N Engl J Med 2001;345:1359–67.
2. Preiser J, Devos P, Ruiz-Santana S, et al. A prospective randomised multi-centre controlled trial on tight glucose control by intensive insulin therapy in adult intensive care units: the Glucontrol study. Intensive Care Med 2009;35:1738–48.
3. Finfer S, Chittock D, Su S, et al. Intensive versus conventional glucose control in critically ill patients. N Engl J Med 2009;360:1283–97.
4. Griesdale D, de Souza R, van Dam R, et al. Intensive insulin therapy and mortality among critically ill patients: a meta-analysis including NICE-SUGAR study data. CMAJ 2009;180:821–7.
5. Wiener RS, Wiener DC, Larson RJ. Benefits and risks of tight glucose control in critically ill adults: a meta-analysis. JAMA 2008;300:933–44.
6. Moghissi E, Korytkowski M, DiNardo M, et al. American Association of Clinical Endocrinologists and American Diabetes Association consensus statement on inpatient glycemic control. Diabetes Care 2009;32(6):1119–31.
7. American Diabetes Association. Standards of medical care in diabetes—2012. Diabetes Care 2012;35:S11–63.
8. Kitabchi A, Umpierrez G, Murphy M, et al. Management of hyperglycemic crises in patients with diabetes. Diabetes Care 2001;24:131–53.
9. Malmberg K, the DIGAMI Study Group. Prospective randomized study of intensive insulin treatment on long-term survival after acute myocardial infarction in patients with diabetes mellitus. BMJ 1997;314:1512–5.
10. Trence D, Kelly J, Hirsch I. The rationale and management of hyperglycemia for in-patients with cardiovascular disease: time for change. J Clin Endocrinol Metab 2003;88:2430–7.
11. Davidson PC, Steed RD, Bode BW. Glucommander: a computer-directed intravenous insulin system shown to be safe, simple, and effective in 120,618 h of operation. Diabetes Care 2005;28:2418–23.
12. Cole R, Ash J. Glucose or carbohydrate supply during continuous intravenous insulin administration in the intensive care unit. Diabetes Technol Ther 2008;10:50.
13. Steil G, Deiss D, Shih J, et al. Intensive care unit insulin delivery algorithms: why so many? How to choose? J Diabetes Sci Technol 2009;3:125–40.
14. Yamashita S, Ng E, Brommecker F, et al. Implementation of the Glucommander method of adjusting insulin infusions in critically ill patients. Can J Hosp Pharm 2011;64:333–9.
15. Juneja R, Roudebush C, Kumar N, et al. Utilization of a computerized intravenous insulin infusion program to control blood glucose in the intensive care unit. Diabetes Technol Ther 2007;9:232–40.
16. Lee J, Fortlage D, Box K, et al. Computerized insulin infusion programs are safe and effective in the burn intensive care unit. J Burn Care Res 2012;33:e114–9.
17. Dortch M, Mowery N, Ozdas A, et al. A computerized insulin infusion titration protocol improves glucose control with less hypoglycemia compared to a manual titration protocol in a trauma intensive care unit. J Parenter Enteral Nutr 2008;32:18–27.

18. Mann E, Jones J, Wolf S, et al. Computer decision support software safely improves glycemic control in the burn intensive care unit: a randomized controlled clinical study. J Burn Care Res 2011;32:246–55.

19. Furnary A, Wu Y. Clinical effects of hyperglycemia in the cardiac surgery population: the Portland Diabetic Project. Endocr Pract 2006;12(Suppl 3):22–6.

20. Providence Health and Services. Portland Diabetes Project: frequently asked questions. Available at: http://oregon.providence.org/patients/healthconditionscare/portland-diabetes-protocols/Pages/proprietaryhealtharticlelanding.aspx?&TemplateName=Portland+Diabetes+Project+Frequently+Asked+Questions&TemplateType=PropietaryHealthArticle. Accessed September 28, 2012.

21. Goldberg P, Siegel M, Sherwin R, et al. Implementation of a safe and effective insulin infusion protocol in a medical intensive care unit. Diabetes Care 2004; 27:461–7.

Perioperative Care of Patients with Diabetes

Celia M. Levesque, RN, MSN, NP-C, CNS-BC, BC-ADM, CDE

KEYWORDS

- Diabetes • Surgery • Diabetes medications • Hyperglycemia • Hypoglycemia

KEY POINTS

- Patients with diabetes undergo surgery more often than those without diabetes.
- Surgical patients with diabetes have a higher rate of morbidity and longer hospital stays than patients without diabetes.
- An optimal perioperative plan of care for patients with diabetes is vital to reduce risk for acute complications secondary to poor glucose control.

INTRODUCTION

Diabetes is present in 8.3% of the United States population,[1] but its prevalence in surgical patients is 15%–20%.[2] Most of the surgical patients with diabetes are not hospitalized before arriving for surgery, but their postsurgical course is clearly affected by the disease. Surgical patients with diabetes have a higher rate of morbidity and longer hospital stays than patients without diabetes.[3] Patients with diabetes also have a 50% higher risk of surgery-related mortality than those without diabetes.[4] Surgical site infection rates are 2 to 3 times higher in patients with diabetes, and wound healing is often suboptimal.[4] Although there are no published studies to support one perioperative diabetes management protocol over another, use of a standardized protocol has been found to be safe and effective.[5] This article discusses the effects of surgery on blood glucose, preoperative assessment of the patient with diabetes, blood glucose targets during the perioperative period, and adjustment of diabetes medications during the perioperative period.

EFFECTS OF SURGERY ON BLOOD GLUCOSE

Surgery increases the release of catabolic hormones (epinephrine, glucagon, cortisol, and growth hormone) and inflammatory cytokines (interleukin-6 and tumor necrosis

Disclosure: The author has no relationship with a commercial company that has a direct financial interest in the subject matter or materials discussed in the article or with a company making a competing product.
Department of Endocrine Neoplasia and Hormonal Disorders, The University of Texas MD Anderson Cancer Center, PO Box 301402, Unit 1461, Houston, TX 77230-1402, USA
E-mail address: clevesqu@mdanderson.org

factor-α) and decreases the release of anabolic hormones, especially insulin, which leads to insulin resistance and hyperglycemia.[3,4] Some patients without a history of diabetes will have transient hyperglycemia after surgery. Patients with type 1 diabetes do not produce insulin and are unable to respond to the increased demand for insulin during and after surgery. They are at high risk for diabetic ketoacidosis development if insulin is not replaced during the perioperative period. Patients with type 2 diabetes produce variable amounts of insulin, have a relative insulin deficiency secondary to insulin resistance, and have a reduced ability to respond to the increased demand for insulin during and after surgery. Although patients with type 2 diabetes have a lower risk of diabetic ketoacidosis development compared with those with type 1 diabetes, they also need careful assessment and monitoring during the perioperative period.

ASSESSMENT BEFORE SURGERY

If the surgery is elective, a thorough assessment should be performed and a plan implemented to minimize comorbid risk factors. A complete diabetes history, including diabetes medication history, diet history, and review of the blood glucose logbook, should be taken and a physical examination performed. Patients with diabetes should be assessed for a history of poor glucose control, frequent or severe hypoglycemia, hypoglycemia unawareness, diabetic ketoacidosis, hyperglycemic hyperosmolar states, cardiovascular disease, cerebrovascular disease, hypertension, chronic kidney disease, peripheral vascular disease, autonomic neuropathy, and peripheral neuropathy. Elevated glycated hemoglobin (HbA1c) levels are associated with adverse surgical outcomes.[3] The target HbA1c level for a patient depends on his or her risk for hypoglycemia. Cardiac, renal, and peripheral nerve function should be assessed. Preoperative testing should include electrocardiography and measurements of a metabolic panel, electrolytes, and HbA1c. The type of anesthesia, type of surgery (minor or major), the start and end times of surgery, the amount of time the patient will be fasting, the type of diet that will be ordered after surgery, and the type of intravenous fluids that will be administered all should be ascertained. If time allows, the level of HbA1c should be reduced to less than 7% because this level is associated with a lower incidence of postoperative infection.[6]

BLOOD GLUCOSE TARGET IN THE PERIOPERATIVE PERIOD

The blood glucose target during the perioperative period is a matter of debate. Van den Berghe and colleagues[7] found reductions in surgery-related morbidity and mortality in surgical intensive care patients randomly assigned to the group with the goal of achieving blood glucose levels of 80–110 mg/dL compared with the conventional goal group who had the goal of achieving blood glucose levels of 180–200 mg/dL. The NICE-SUGAR (Normoglycemia in Intensive Care Evaluation-Survival Using Glucose Algorithm Regulation) study found that patients in the intensive arm of the study (glucose goal of 81–108 mg/dL) had higher rates of severe hypoglycemia and mortality than the control group (glucose goal of <180 mg/dL).[8] The American Association of Clinical Endocrinologists and the American Diabetes Association published a consensus statement regarding inpatient glycemic control, although it was not specific to surgical patients with diabetes.[9] They recommended that insulin therapy be initiated in patients with blood glucose levels greater than 180 mg/dL, with a target of maintaining a glucose range of 140–180 mg/dL for most critically ill patients. For most non–critically ill patients, they recommended a premeal blood glucose target of less than 140 mg/dL and a random blood glucose target less than 180 mg/dL. They recommended scheduled subcutaneous insulin replacement with basal, nutritional, and correction components rather than sliding-scale insulin therapy.

The Society for Ambulatory Anesthesia developed a consensus statement regarding care for patients with diabetes undergoing ambulatory surgery.[10] The organization found insufficient data to recommend blood glucose or HbA1c levels above which elective surgery should be postponed; however, the statement says that surgery should be postponed if the patient has complications of hyperglycemia, including dehydration, ketoacidosis, and hyperosmolar nonketotic states. They suggested maintaining an intraoperative blood glucose level of less than 180 mg/dL for most patients, but the goal level is dependent on factors such as the duration of surgery, invasiveness of the procedure, type of anesthesia, duration of fasting, and diabetes medication regimen before the procedure. They recommended that patients with a previous history of poorly controlled diabetes maintain their preoperative baseline values rather than try to normalize the blood glucose, because such patients have an altered counter-regulatory response, which leads to symptoms of hypoglycemia when the blood glucose level is normal and because acute reduction in blood glucose can cause an oxidative stress response, which increases the risk of perioperative morbidity and mortality.

ADJUSTMENT OF NONINSULIN DIABETES MEDICATIONS

If a patient is not taking any diabetes medications before surgery, blood glucose levels should be measured before and after surgery. Hyperglycemia can be treated with rapid- or short-acting insulin as needed. Taking sulfonylureas increases insulin secretion for 24 hours or more and can cause hypoglycemia. If a patient is taking a sulfonylurea before surgery and is eating normally, the drug can be administered the day before surgery. The dose may be reduced or omitted if the patient's diet is restricted the day before surgery. Sulfonylureas should be omitted the day of surgery and restarted when the patient is eating well.

Meglitinides also increase insulin secretion but last for a shorter period. They can cause hypoglycemia, although the risk is smaller than that arising from sulfonylurea use. Meglitinides may be given with each meal the day before surgery but need to be omitted on the day of surgery. They may be restarted once the patient is eating well.

Thiazolidinediones do not cause insulin secretion and therefore do not cause hypoglycemia. They may be given the day before surgery but will be withheld while the patient is prohibited from oral intake.

Biguanides inhibit liver glucose production and augment peripheral glucose uptake. They do not increase insulin secretion or, consequently, hypoglycemia; however, if lactic acidosis develops, biguanides may exacerbate the condition. Biguanides may be given the day before surgery but should be withheld the day of surgery and restarted when good renal function is verified after surgery and the patient is eating. Biguanides are not used in male patients with a creatinine level of 1.5 mg/dL or higher, female patients with a creatinine level of 1.4 mg/dL or higher, or patients with significant liver disease or heart failure.

Other agents that should be withheld on the day of surgery are α-glycosidase inhibitors, incretin mimics, and dipeptidyl peptidase-4 inhibitors. Amylin agonists can be administered on the day of surgery, but only with a meal. All these agents can be resumed once the patient is eating well. See **Table 1** for oral diabetes medications, **Table 2** for insulins, and **Table 3** for noninsulin injectable medications and their implications for surgery. **Table 4** summarizes recommendations for the adjustment of injectable diabetes medications on the day before surgery.

Table 1
Oral diabetes medications

Medication Names Generic (Trademark)	Mechanism of Action	Surgery Implication
Sulfonylureas: Glimepiride (Amaryl) Glipizide (Glucotrol, Glucotrol XL) Glyburide (Diabeta, Glynase PresTab, Micronase)	Increase insulin secretion in people with capacity to produce insulin; may also decrease the rate of hepatic glucose production, and increase insulin receptor sensitivity and the number of insulin receptors	Sulfonylureas may need to be reduced or omitted the day before surgery depending on the diet prescribed. They should not be used in patients who are fasting because of the increased risk of hypoglycemia
Meglitinides: Nateglinide (Starlix) Repaglinide (Prandin)	Increase insulin secretion by binding to K+ channels on β islet cells. Repaglinide is metabolized by the liver enzymes CYP3A4 and CYP2C8. Nateglinide is metabolized by hepatic CYP450 CYP2C9 (70%) and CYP3A4 (30%)	Meglitinides are taken immediately before eating a meal and therefore should not be used in patients who are fasting for surgery
Thiazolidinediones: Pioglitazone (Actos) Rosiglitizone (Avandia)	Improve target cell response to insulin; decrease hepatic gluconeogenesis. Metabolized to active metabolites by hepatic CYP2C8 and CYP34A	Thiazolidinediones do not cause hypoglycemia and therefore can be given when the patient is not on nothing-by-mouth status
Biguanides: Metformin (Glucophage, Glucophage XR, Glumetza, Fortamet, Riomet)	Decrease hepatic glucose production and gastrointestinal glucose absorption; increase target cell insulin sensitivity	Biguanides should not be used in female patients with a creatinine level ≥ 1.4 mg/dL or male patients with a creatinine level ≥1.5 mg/dL. Biguanides should be withheld the day of surgery not restarted until good renal function has been verified by lab analysis and the patient is eating well
Alpha glucosidase inhibitors: Acarbose (Precose) Miglitol (Glyset)	Delay gastrointestinal absorption of carbohydrate	Alpha glucosidase inhibitors are taken just before meals. They can be given once the patient begins to eat meals after surgery
Dipeptidyl peptidase-4 inhibitors: Sitagliptin phosphate (Januvia) Saxagliptin (Onglyza) Linagliptin (Tradjenta)	Increase and prolong incretin hormone activity, which is inactivated by dipeptidyl peptidase-4 activity; metabolism limited, primarily by CYP3A4	Dipeptidyl peptidase-4 inhibitors do not cause hypoglycemia. They can be given when the patient is not on nothing-by-mouth status

Abbreviation: CY, Cytochrome.

Table 2
Insulin

Medication Names Generic (Trademark)	Onset	Peak	Duration	Surgery Implication
Aspart (Novolog) Lispro (Humalog) Glulisine (Apidra)	15 min	90 min	2–4 h	Used as a bolus insulin to treat hyperglycemia
Regular (Humulin R, Novolin R, Relion R)	30–60 min	2–4 h	6–8 h	Used as a bolus insulin for hyperglycemia; can be given intravenously or subcutaneously. If given subcutaneously, take care not to give too frequently, as this can result in hypoglycemia
NPH (Humulin N, Novolin N, Relion N)	2–4 h	4–12 h	12–18 h	NPH has a peak effect. Either the dose may need to be reduced or the insulin discontinued for surgery
Detemir (Levemir) Glargine (Lantus)	4–6 h	Peakless	16–24 h	If the patient is fasting for a prolonged time, the basal insulin requirement will be reduced. Many patients use basal insulin to cover food requirements and will need a dose reduction for surgery.

Table 3
Noninsulin injectable diabetes medications

Medication Names Generic (Trademark)	Mechanism of Action	Surgery Implication
Incretin mimetics: Exenatide (Byetta) Exenatide extended release (Bydureon) Liraglutide (Victoza)	Synthetic analogs of exendin-4, a gila monster salivary polypeptide that mimics incretin and promotes insulin secretion, suppresses glucagon, and slows gastric emptying	Incretin mimetics do not produce hypoglycemia. They are given on days when the patient is going to eat meals. They cause delayed gastric emptying and can cause nausea
Amylin agonists: Pramlintide (Symlin)	Synthetic analogs of the polypeptide pancreatic hormone amylin, which slows gastric emptying, suppresses glucagon, and regulates appetite	Amylin agonists are given immediately before meals with rapid-acting insulin for the meal. They would not be given unless the patient is eating a meal

INSULIN THERAPY IN SURGERY PATIENTS WITH DIABETES

Insulin replacement during the perioperative period should be administered to mimic normal physiologic insulin release (basal/bolus), with the goal of avoiding hypoglycemia and severe hyperglycemia. The purpose of basal insulin is to maintain adequate blood glucose control between meals. Basal insulin can include insulin detemir, insulin glargine, neutral protamine Hagedorn (NPH) insulin, or the basal rate of an insulin pump. Patients with type 2 diabetes may not require basal insulin replacement to avoid diabetic ketoacidosis; however, replacement is necessary in patients with type 1 diabetes. The basal insulin dose may need to be decreased for surgery if the patient reports that hypoglycemia occurs when a meal is missed or delayed, if the patient will be missing more than one meal for surgery, or if the patient's diet is restricted preoperatively.

Bolus insulin includes meal and correctional doses. Meal insulin is given with food to maintain target blood glucose after eating. Correction insulin is given to bring an elevated blood glucose level down to the target range. The insulin used to maintain postprandial insulin levels or correct hyperglycemia may be rapid-acting insulin (such as insulin aspart, insulin glulisine, and insulin lispro) or short-acting insulin (such as regular insulin).

Because the patient is not eating during surgery, the rapid- or short-acting insulin is only used for correction of hyperglycemia. On the day before surgery and again once the patient resumes eating meals, short- or rapid-acting insulin is given with food. Intravenous bolus doses of regular insulin are not recommended because its short duration of action (30–40 minutes) causes wide fluctuations in the blood glucose level.[10] For patients who are not in critical condition, the American Association of Clinical Endocrinologists/American Diabetes Association consensus statement recommends subcutaneous administration of insulin; however, very short dose intervals should be avoided because they can lead to hypoglycemia.[9]

INSULIN THERAPY IN LONG OR COMPLEX SURGICAL PROCEDURES

Intravenous insulin is preferred to subcutaneous insulin during long or complex procedures because tissue perfusion may be unpredictable. The half-life of intravenous regular insulin is 5–10 minutes, allowing for precise dose administration and titration

Table 4
Recommendations for perioperative adjustment of diabetes medications

Medication	Recommendations: Evening Before Surgery	Recommendations: Day of Surgery
Sulfonylureas	Withhold	Withhold
Meglitinides	Give with meals	Withhold while patient status is nothing by mouth
Thiazolidinediones	Give	Withhold while patient status is nothing by mouth
Biguanides	Give	Withhold until the postoperative creatinine level is <1.4 mg/dL in female patients and <1.5 mg/dL in male patients and the patient resumes eating meals
Alpha glucosidase inhibitors	Give with meals	Withhold
Dipeptidyl peptidase-4 inhibitors	Give	Withhold
Incretin mimetics	Give	Withhold
Amylin agonists	Give with meals	Withhold
Rapid-Acting insulin	Give usual dose for food and hyperglycemia treatment	Use only for corrections of hyperglycemia
Short-Acting insulin	Give usual dose for food and hyperglycemia treatment	Use only for corrections of hyperglycemia
Intermediate-Acting insulin	Give usual dose in the morning; may need a reduced dose the evening before surgery	Give 50%–75% of dose before surgery
Pre-mixed insulin	Give usual dose	Switch to a basal/bolus method
Long-Acting insulin	Give usual dose	Type 1 diabetes: give 50% of usual dose Type 2 diabetes: withhold or give 50% of usual dose
Insulin pump	Give usual dose	If discontinuing, give 50% of the total basal dose as a long-acting insulin before surgery. Check blood glucose every 1–2 h and give rapid-acting insulin for correction of hyperglycemia, being careful not to stack the insulin doses. If patient remains on pump: have him or her set a temporary basal rate at 50%–80% of the usual rate. Make sure the pump site is intact and out of the way of the planned surgical site and that the pump site is less than 3 days old. Check blood glucose every 1–2 h and give rapid-acting insulin for correction of hyperglycemia, being careful not to stack the insulin doses.

based on the blood glucose level. The insulin infusion should be started early in the morning the day of surgery to allow time to achieve the target blood glucose level. If a patient is receiving basal insulin before surgery, the infusion should not be stopped before subcutaneous basal insulin is resumed, especially if the patient has type 1 diabetes.[10]

SLIDING-SCALE SHORT-ACTING OR RAPID-ACTING INSULIN

Sliding-scale insulin regimens, when used alone, may produce widely fluctuating blood glucose levels because doses are given only when the patient's blood glucose level is high. Patients with type 1 diabetes should never be placed on a sliding-scale insulin regimen alone; they must be prescribed basal insulin as well.[9]

DAY OF SURGERY

Surgery should be scheduled in the morning so the patient does not miss more than one meal, which would increase the risk of catabolism. If the patient misses more than one meal, fluid replacement may be needed to prevent gluconeogenesis, lipolysis, ketogenesis, and proteolysis and to maintain euvolemia and serum electrolyte levels. The patient's blood glucose level should be tested at the time of his or her arrival for surgery, every 1–2 hours during surgery, and in the immediate postoperative period.[4] Again, **Table 4** summarizes recommendations for adjustment of diabetes medications on the day of surgery.

Basal insulin, if needed, should be given in the morning of surgery at the usual prescribed time. If applicable, pump use should continue until basal insulin has been injected. If the patient is going to wear the insulin pump during surgery, the pump infusion site should not interfere with the surgery and be less than 3 days old.

If the patient's blood glucose level is less than 70 mg/dL, 20–50 mL of intravenous 50% dextrose (10–25 g) may be given. If there is no intravenous access, 1 mg of glucagon may be administered via intramuscular injection. If the patient is not prohibited from oral intake, he or she may be given 15 g of carbohydrate by mouth in the form of a clear liquid. The caregiver should recheck the patient's blood glucose level every 15 minutes and repeat the treatment until it exceeds 70 mg/dL.

POSTOPERATIVE CARE

Most patients can resume their usual medication regimen after surgery. However, sulfonylureas and meglitinides should not be restarted until the patient is eating well because of the risk of hypoglycemia. Metformin should not be restarted until good renal function is verified and the patient is confirmed to be neither acidotic nor have significant liver disease or heart failure that would predispose the patient to acidosis. Thiazolidinediones should not be restarted if congestive heart failure, significant fluid retention, or significant liver dysfunction develop.

If the patient is started on tube feeding, subcutaneous insulin will probably be needed. The insulin dose will depend on the amount of carbohydrate in the tube feeding. If the patient is receiving total parenteral nutrition, he or she will probably need regular insulin as well. If the patient is on a clear liquid diet, his or her meals may contain little carbohydrate (if the patient chooses broth, diet Jello-O, diet soda, and similar items) or a lot of carbohydrate (if the patient chooses juices, regular soda, regular Jello-O, and so on). The prescriber should interview the patient to ascertain the amount of carbohydrate that the patient will consume before ordering prandial insulin.

SUMMARY

There are no strong, randomized research trials supporting a single approach to perioperative care of patients with diabetes. The literature does, however, support performing a thorough preoperative assessment, choosing safe glucose targets, and, if possible, minimizing risk factors that increase the risk of postoperative complications. When developing a hospital perioperative protocol, one should know how each class of diabetes medication works and how to adjust the dose before, during, and after surgery. Maintaining the blood glucose level in the target range and resuming nutrition as quickly as possible reduce the risk of acute complications such as hypoglycemia, significant hyperglycemia, diabetic ketoacidosis, hyperosmolar hyperglycemic state, electrolyte imbalances, and dehydration.

ACKNOWLEDGMENTS

The author acknowledges the Scientific Editing Department at MD Anderson Hospital for reviewing and editing the manuscript.

REFERENCES

1. Centers for Disease Control and Prevention. 2011 National Diabetes Fact Sheet. Available at: http://www.dcd.gov/diabetes/pubs/estimates11htm. Accessed April 12, 2012.
2. Power M, Ostrow L. Preoperative diabetes management protocol for adult outpatients. J Perianesth Nurs 2008;23:371–8.
3. Meneghini L. Perioperative management of diabetes: translating evidence into practice. Cleve Clin J Med 2009;76:S53–9.
4. Dhatanya K, Levy N, Kilvert A, et al. Diabetes UK position statements and care recommendations: NHS diabetes guideline for the perioperative management of the adult patient with diabetes. Diabet Med 2012;29:420–33.
5. DiNardo M, Donihi A, Forte P, et al. Standardized glycemic management and perioperative glycemic outcomes in patients with diabetes mellitus who undergo same-day surgery. Endocr Pract 2011;17:404–11.
6. Dronge A, Perkal M, Kancir S, et al. Long-term glycemic control and postoperative infectious complications. Arch Surg 2006;141(4):375.
7. Van den Berghe G, Wouters P, Weekers F, et al. Intensive insulin therapy in the critically ill patients. N Engl J Med 2001;345:1359–67.
8. NICE-SUGAR Study Investigators. Intensive vs conventional glucose control in critically ill patients. N Engl J Med 2009;360:1283–97.
9. Moghissi E, Korytkowsi M, DiNardo M, et al. American Association of Clinical Endocrinologists and American diabetes Association consensus statement on inpatient glycemic control. Diabetes Care 2009;32:1119–31.
10. Joshi G, Chung F, Vann M, et al. Society for Ambulatory Anesthesia consensus statement on perioperative blood glucose management in diabetic patients undergoing ambulatory surgery. In: International Anesthesia Research Society. 2010. Available at: http://anesthesia-analgesia.org/content/early/2010/10/01/ANE.0b013e3181f9c288.full.pdf. Accessed April 12, 2012.

Hyperglycemic Management After Solid Organ Transplantation

Johnny L. Rollins, RN, MSN, ANP-C

KEYWORDS

- New-onset diabetes after transplantation • Posttransplant diabetes mellitus
- Steroid-induced hyperglycemia • Diabetes • Transplant surgery • Hyperglycemia

KEY POINTS

- Hyperglycemia increases risks for wound infections and poor healing times.
- Hyperglycemia increases risks for graft rejection and graft loss.
- Untreated hyperglycemia increases risks for advancement to diabetes mellitus.
- Controlling hyperglycemia can reduce the prevalence of new-onset diabetes after transplantation.

INTRODUCTION

Evidence-based medicine heightened the medical community's consciousness of improving inpatient glycemic control. Hyperglycemia increases a patient's risk for graft failure and rejection, prolongs hospital stay, and increases the risk of infection and poor wound healing.[1–4] Impaired insulin production and/or increased insulin resistance results in hyperglycemia,[2,5] which results in β-cell dysfunction, resulting diabetes.[6–8]

It is critical that glucose levels are managed during all aspects of the patient's hospitalization; pre-operatively, intraoperatively and postoperatively. The pancreatic β cells can be protected and islet function preserved with early interventions to control the severe hyperglycemia associated with solid organ transplantation.[4] Hyperglycemia is an extremely common complication with solid organ transplantation.[1–10] Multiple factors are associated with hyperglycemia, including stress of surgery, pain, high-dose glucocorticoids (often called *steroids*), immunosuppressive therapies, and nutrition. Hecking and colleagues[4] reported a strong effect on glucose levels from the

Disclosure: The author has no relationship with a commercial company that has a direct financial interest in the subject matter or materials discussed in the article or with a company making a competing product.
Department of Endocrine Neoplasia and Hormonal Disorders, The University of Texas MD Anderson Cancer Center, 1400 Pressler Street, Unit 1461, Houston, TX 77030, USA
E-mail address: jlrollin@mdanderson.org

Crit Care Nurs Clin N Am 25 (2013) 31–38
http://dx.doi.org/10.1016/j.ccell.2012.11.013
0899-5885/13/$ – see front matter © 2013 Elsevier Inc. All rights reserved.

synergistic effects of calcineurin inhibitors, steroids, and immunosuppressive medications.

CURRENT LITERATURE

A review of general organ transplant literature chronicles the medical community movements toward a major lifelong complication. Many transplant physicians expect hyperglycemia after organ transplantation and do not treat their patients until glucose levels are significantly out of control, usually greater 250 mg/dL. However, based on recent research and the increase in patient survival after transplant, the age-old hyperglycemia related to steroids has mutated into the development of new-onset diabetes after transplantation (NODAT).[1–6] The heightened awareness of NODAT has not generated a consensus on the definition of the condition.[10] The American Diabetes Association (ADA) states that random glucose levels greater than 200 mg/dL with hyperglycemic symptoms are diagnostic for diabetes.

Patients with uncontrolled and/or untreated hyperglycemia are at serious risk for developing diabetes.[7] According to Davidson and colleagues,[10] diabetes and impaired glucose tolerance are common problems associated with solid organ transplantation, and the development of NODAT is more than 50% in some studies. Multiple studies show that hyperglycemia and uncontrolled diabetes mellitus result in serious postoperative complications.[10] Posttransplant glucose control is critical for patient survival.[2–4] Uncontrolled hyperglycemia is associated with graft failure, predisposing patients to increased risks of morbidity and mortality.[1–4,6,8–10] Undermanaged hyperglycemia predisposes patients to pancreatic stress with slow deterioration of islet cells, resulting in pancreatic β-cell dysfunction.[11] Diabetes is associated heart disease, kidney disease, stroke, loss of limbs, and death.[7]

Postoperative solid organ transplantation hyperglycemia must be managed aggressively and promptly. Early interventions for pancreatic β-cell rest and islet cell protection can reduce the escalation toward NODAT.[2,4]

PATHOLOGY

Glucose levels greater than 200 mg/dL are classified as hyperglycemia using the ADA criteria and current transplant publications and studies.[1–5,8–11] Multiple factors increase the patient's hyperglycemic risk after organ transplantation: pain, steroids, calcineurin inhibitors, and nutrition. Hyperglycemia during surgery is strong indicator for postoperative complications.[12] Immediately postoperatively, the body is under a vast amount of stress related to the surgery. Stress has a wide range of physical effects on the human body. The endocrine response to increased physiologic stress results in activation of the adrenal cortex.[13] This activation results in release of corticosteroids. The release of these corticosteroids produces hyperglycemia and insulin resistance.[13,14]

The patient is given intravenous glucocorticoids preoperatively, which will cause hyperglycemia.[14] Steroids have a direct impact on the pancreatic β cells by directly inhibiting insulin release.[11,13] These glucocorticoids are linked to decreased insulin uptake and increased hepatic glucose production requiring increased prandial insulin doses.[13] Lansang and Hustak[13] reported glucose levels greater than 200 mg/dL 2 hours after eating in patients with a normal fasting plasma glucose level while on steroids. Patients typically receive a bolus dose of steroids before transplant surgery, and a tapering regimen is initiated after completion. Glucocorticoids are used in combination with other immunosuppressive medications to prevent graft rejection.

Calcineurin inhibitors are primarily used for immunosuppression posttransplant to prevent graft rejection. Cyclosporine and tacrolimus have been linked to the development of NODAT.[5] Tacrolimus is dose-dependent, with higher blood levels correlated with higher glucose levels.[10] Patients who were transitioned to cyclosporine no longer required insulin therapy.[8,10]

DIAGNOSIS AND TREATMENT

Currently no consensus exists on the diagnosis of NODAT, and consequently no specific standardized treatment algorithms exist for this condition. The literature is flooded with the ongoing debate in the medical community about glucose control inside the hospital and especially regarding postsurgical and critically ill patients. The transplant literature recommends that all patients undergo glucose monitoring after solid organ transplantation.[10] Frequency of testing is debatable, and currently no clear guidelines exist. The 2003 International Consensus Guidelines for NODAT recommended that fasting plasma glucose levels be monitored every morning with at least 8 hours of no caloric intake.[10] However, no recommendations are noted for inpatient monitoring. Chakkera and colleagues[9] recommended monitoring glucose levels every 6 to 8 hours after kidney transplantation.

Treatment Goals

The current recommendation is to follow the American Association of Clinical Endocrinologists (AACE) and the ADA consensus statement regarding inpatient glycemic control.[10] Glucose target goals should be no less than 110 mg/dL and no higher than 180 mg/dL. Critically ill patients should maintain glucose levels on the upper limits of this goal, with a target ranging from 140 to 180 mg/dL. The goals are to avoid postoperative hypoglycemia and hyperglycemia. Once the patient is stable and no longer in the critical care unit, care should focus on tighter glucose management, with the targeted goal ranging from 110 to 140 mg/dL. Glucose readings greater than 180 mg/dL should be unacceptable in a stable recovering patient.

Intensive Care

Immediately on arrival in the intensive care unit, patients should be started on intensive glucose monitoring.[12] During this critical time, glucose management and control are as important as starting patients on immunosuppressive medications. Hyperglycemia during the immediate postoperative period is an independent predictor of morbidity and mortality in patients with and without a diagnosis of diabetes.[12] Continuous insulin infusions (CIIs) should be the preferred drug treatment during the immediate the postoperative period. Initiation of CIIs in patients with a glucose level greater then 180 mg/dL should be the standard of care for all patients after solid organ transplantation surgery. The goal is to decrease pancreatic β-cell stress and workload, therefore allowing improved pancreatic β-cell function during the home recovery period.[4]

Insulin drips are an extremely safe and effective method of controlling hyperglycemia with minimal hypoglycemic events, if the protocols can factor the rate of glucose levels decreasing.[13] Intensive glucose monitoring during CII and frequent titration of the drip rate are required. The half-life of intravenous insulin is extremely short, and when the CII is stopped, the insulin is stopped and rapidly cleared from the patient's system, which is in glaring contrast to subcutaneous insulin injections. Once the patient receives the subcutaneous insulin injection, it cannot be stopped if the patient starts experiencing hypoglycemia. Furthermore, depending on the type of insulin, it could remain in the system for up to 24 hours or longer in patients with decreased renal function or impaired liver function. These effects could require additional interventions, such as glucose infusions or glucagon injections.

Adverse Effects

Glucose instability

Although CII is a safe and effective practice in managing hyperglycemia, especially immediately during the postoperative period or during high stress doses of steroids, patients may require a subcutaneous injection if they are tolerating oral intake and are on a diet.[13,15] Caloric intake coupled with high-dose steroids has the potential to double the glucose level after a meal.[13] CII protocols for glucose testing are usually every 1 hour and if stable maybe every 2 to 3 hours.

Case study

Mr Smith is currently on a CII drip at 2.25 U/h, with a stable glucose trend ranging from 140 to 150 mg/dL over the last 4 hours. He received his 125 mg dose of methylprednisolone intravenously approximately 3 hours previously and is eating a regular diet. His glucose level after his meal is now 360 mg/dL.

The CII protocol for a patient such as Mr Smith recommends administering an intravenous bolus dose of insulin and increasing the drip rate, and repeating the glucose test in 1 hour. The nurse will spend the next 3 to 5 hours chasing the glucose and adjusting the drip rate. Overcorrection is a possible complication in this case, which will result in hypoglycemia and stopping the insulin infusion. This action will result in rebound hyperglycemia: the "roller coaster effect."

The roller coaster effect is a vicious cycle of highs and lows in the patient's glucose trends. A prandial or mealtime dose of insulin will decrease the severe postprandial hyperglycemia effect. With the initiation of the subcutaneous prandial insulin, postprandial glucose excursions will stabilize and the roller coaster effect will be avoided.

A smooth transition from insulin infusion therapy to subcutaneous insulin therapy is needed. Using the 70% rule for transition from intravenous to subcutaneous insulin is a safe starting point; the conversion calculation is provided in **Fig. 1**. If this transition is not performed effectively, the patient will experience the roller coaster effect. Intravenous insulin has an extremely short half-life (<10 minutes), and when the CII drip is turned off, the glucose levels begin to escalate. The subcutaneous and CII therapies must overlap to avoid the roller coaster effect. A good method is to administer a dose of basal insulin and wait at least 2 hour before discontinuing the CII drip. **Fig. 2** provides the calculation for multiple daily injections (MDIs) for the basal and prandial insulin dose.

Conversion formula from CII to SQ insulin

70% Rule

Total IV insulin dose for 24 h X 70% = Total daily insulin dose for SQ injections

CII = 225 units   SQ = 157.5 units (158 units)

Fig. 1. Conversion formula from CII to subcutaneous insulin. IV, intravenous; SQ, subcutaneous.

Calculation for MDI

60-40 Rule

40% of the Total daily insulin dose for SQ injections will be basal insulin
60% of the Total daily insulin dose for SQ injections will be prandial insulin

TDD = 158 units   Basal = 63.2 units (63 units)   Prandial = 94.8 units (95 units)

Fig. 2. Calculation for multiple daily injections. TTD, total daily dose.

Once the patient is stabilized and tolerating oral intake, and the diet is advanced, transitioning to glucose testing before meals and at bedtime is recommended. Some recommendations suggest that monitoring glucose levels 1 to 2 hours post-prandial is beneficial in evaluating treatment regimens.[13] However, glucose testing must occur in concert with treatment interventions. Another complication of steroid therapy is that it makes the patient hungry, and they tend to crave simple sugars and carbohydrates, resulting in higher postprandial glucose loads.[13] Insulin tends to improve glucose levels when injected. The 60/40 rule, patients require more prandial insulin coverage than basal insulin coverage (see **Fig. 2**).

Dependency
All steroids have an effect on glucose levels. **Table 1** provides a list of commonly used steroids and their biologic half-lives. During critical illness, periods of high stress, and cycles of high-dose steroids, oral medications might not the best drug choice for glucose control. Using sulfonylurea oral medications will result in a greater workload for pancreatic β cells, resulting in β-cell dysfunction. Meglitinides are a slightly better choice than sulfonylureas; they have a shorter duration of workload on the pancreatic β cell. However, the steroid effect related to postprandial hyperglycemia might not be controlled with these short-acting medications. In immunosuppressed patients in the immediate posttransplant period thiazolidinediones might not be effective because of their long time of onset. Metformin is an excellent drug and is one of the first-line medication recommendations by the ADA and AACE for glycemic control. However, renal function must be monitored closely, and gastrointestinal complications are common. The calcineurin inhibitors can result in acute renal insufficiency and failure. Metformin might not be the preferred drug during the immediate postoperative period. However, 2 or 3 months after organ transplantation if the patient is stable, metformin should be a consideration. What is left? Insulin!

Chronic use
Most people have misinformation about insulin therapy. Many patients have an intense fear that once insulin is started, it can never be stopped, and therefore they do not want insulin. The goal is for pancreatic β-cell rest, and insulin allows these cells to

Table 1		
Commonly used steroids during organ transplantation		
Glucocorticoid	**Approximate Equivalent Dose**	**Half-Life (Biologic) Hours**
Dexamethasone	1 mg	8 h
Methylprednisolone	5 mg	18 h
Prednisone	6.3 mg	18 h
Hydrocortisone	25 mg	36 h

Table 2
Types of insulin, with onset of action, peak, and duration

Name (Brand Name)	Onset of Action	Peak	Duration
Types of Insulin			
Rapid-acting insulin (mealtime insulins or prandial insulins)			
Lispro (Humalog)	<15 min	1–2 h	3–6 h
Aspart (NovoLog)	<15 min	1–2 h	3–6 h
Glulisine (Apidra)	<15 min	1–2 h	3–6 h
Short-acting insulin			
Regular (Novolin R, Humulin R)	30–60 min	2–4 h	6–10 h
Intermediate-acting insulin (basal insulins)			
NPH (Novolin N, Humulin N)	2–4 h	4–8 h	10–18 h
Long-acting insulin (basal insulins)			
Glargine (Lantus)	1–2 h	Usually none	24 h
Detemir (Levemir)	1–2 h	Maybe, usually none	18–24 h

rest. As reported by Hecking and colleagues,[4] early insulin initiation showed an improved pancreatic β-cell function at 3 months and a 73% reduction in NODAT. Insulin is safe and effective, and can be stopped. The patient will not become dependent on insulin. The same cannot be said if oral medications are initiated.

Recommendations

Insulin that is injected works best; it is that simple. Patient education is extremely valuable to help them overcome their fears. All insulin will work to improve glucose levels, and multiple choices of insulin are available. **Table 2** provides a list of the most commonly used prandial and basal insulins, including time of onset, time to peak, and duration. **Fig. 3** depicts a graph of the insulin action on a time line. The goal is to control the patient's glucose while avoiding hypoglycemia in the hospital setting. A few formulas are available for initiating insulin in patients in the outpatient setting, but no clear recommendations exist for the inpatient setting and minimal recommendations exist for initiating subcutaneous insulin in patients receiving high-dose steroids. The

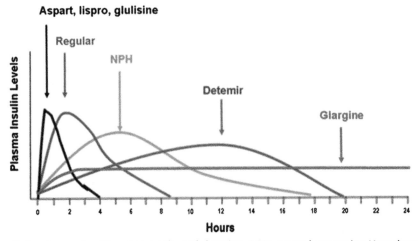

Fig. 3. Insulin graph with onset, peak, and duration. NPH, neutral protamine Hagedorn.

Table 3 High-dose steroids	
Steroid	**Dose**
Dexamethasone	40 mg/d
Methylprednisolone	250 mg/d
Prednisone	300 mg/d

starting dose in the outpatient clinic setting is 0.5 U/kg/d up to 0.75 U/kg/d for the total daily dose (TDD) of insulin, sometimes higher.

Patients receiving high-dose steroids will require more insulin than expected for a TDD of insulin (see **Table 3** for a list of high-dose steroids). A study of patients with cancer on high-dose steroids successfully demonstrated safe and effective guidelines for initiating a high-dose subcutaneous insulin regimen in insulin-naïve patients. The study used a glucose level greater than 250 mg/dL on 2 separate tests before initiating 1.2 U/kg in patients not undergoing concurrent metformin therapy and 1 U/kg in patients currently undergoing metformin therapy (Brady V, Lavis V, unpublished data, 2010). These investigators reported improved glucose management with glucose levels less than 180 mg/dL without significant increase in hypoglycemia using the formula mentioned earlier. Their study also used a 75/25 rule, wherein 75% of the TDD was prandial and the other 25% was basal. The study used detemir as the basal insulin and lispro for prandial insulin.

Lansang and Hustak[13] reported initiating subcutaneous insulin at 0.15 to 0.3 U/kg, and also noted that glucocorticoids would double the insulin requirements. Seggelke and colleagues[14] reported that neutral protamine Hagedorn (NPH) insulin controlled the hyperglycemic effects of methylprednisolone in hospitalized patients. No consensus exists regarding the type of basal insulin initiation; each person is different and every steroid affects patients in many different ways. The best strategy is to start subcutaneous insulin with an MDI regimen, monitor the patient's glucose trends closely, and adjust the insulin doses to keep the glucose range between 110 and 180 mg/dL.

SUMMARY

The author has practiced with the belief that if the pancreatic β cells are able to rest during times of stress, those same cells will maintain their function later in life. Heckling and colleagues[4] showed that this belief is possible. Preserving pancreatic β cells during the hospital stay immediately after solid organ transplantation will decrease the patient's risk of developing NODAT.[8] Controlling postoperative hyperglycemia improves patient outcomes through decreasing the risks of graft failure, surgical wound infections, and death. Oral glucose-lowering medications have the potential to increase the risk of developing NODAT through increasing the workload and stress of the pancreatic β cells. All patients undergoing a solid organ transplant should have glucose levels less than 180 mg/dL during their entire hospital stay. Either CII drips or MDI insulin regimens are necessary for optimal glucose control.

Truly more studies are needed in this arena of medicine. Some new and exciting technologies will emerge in the near future. The hope is that these advances will increase patient safety and decrease the current workload for the bedside nurse. Practitioners should stay tuned in...and remember that insulin can only work if it is injected into the patient. As the author's mentor once said, "vitamin I works well, just use it."

REFERENCES

1. Wilkinson A, Davidson J, Dotta F, et al. Guidelines for the treatment and management of new-onset diabetes after transplantation. Clin Transplant 2005;19:291–8.
2. Chakkera H, Knowler W, Devarapalli Y, et al. Relationship between inpatient hyperglycemia and insulin treatment after kidney transplantation and future new onset diabetes mellitus. Clin J Am Soc Nephrol 2010;5:1669–75.
3. Kasiske B, Snyder J, Gilbertson D, et al. Diabetes mellitus after kidney transplantation in the United States. Am J Transplant 2003;3:178–85.
4. Hecking M, Haidinger M, Döller D, et al. Early basal insulin therapy decreases new-onset diabetes after transplantation. J Am Soc Nephrol 2012;23:739–49.
5. Weir M. Impact of immunosuppressive regimes on posttransplant diabetes mellitus. Transplant Proc 2001;33(Suppl 5A):23S–6S.
6. Viberti G. Diabetes mellitus: a major challenge in transplantation. Transplant Proc 2001;33(Suppl 5A):3S–7S.
7. Dubernard J, Frei U. Introduction. Transplant Proc 2001;33(Suppl 5A):1S–2S.
8. Goldberg P. Comprehensive management of post-transplant diabetes mellitus: from intensive care to home care. Endocrinol Metab Clin North Am 2007;36:907–22.
9. Chakkera H, Weil E, Castro J, et al. Hyperglycemia during the immediate period after kidney transplantation. Clin J Am Soc Nephrol 2009;4:853–9.
10. Davidson J, Wilkinson A, Dantal J, et al. New-onset diabetes after transplant: 2003 International Consensus Guidelines. Transplantation 2003;75(10):SS3–24.
11. Delaunay F, Khan A, Cintra A, et al. Pancreatic beta cells are important targets for the diabetogenic effects of glucocorticoids. J Clin Invest 1997;100(8):2094–8.
12. Lazar H, McDonnell M, Chipkin S, et al. The society of thoracic surgeons practice guideline series: blood glucose management during adult cardiac surgery. Ann Thorac Surg 2009;87:663–9.
13. Lansang M, Hustak L. Glucocorticoid-induced diabetes and adrenal suppression: how to detect and manage them. Cleve Clin J Med 2011;78(11):748–56.
14. Seggelke S, Gibbs J, Draznin B. Pilot study of using neutral protamine hagedorn insulin to counteract the effect of methylprednisolone in hospitalized patients with diabetes. J Hosp Med 2011;6(3):175–6.
15. Hamilton D, Hendricks S, Ihaza E, et al. Glucose management, heart failure and transplantation. Methodist Debakey Cardiovasc J 2009;5(3):12–5.

Use of Noninsulin Antidiabetic Medications in Hospitalized Patients

Cori Kopecky, MSN, RN, OCN*

KEYWORDS

- Diabetes • Diabetes medications • Meglitinides • α-Glucosidase inhibitor
- Dipeptidyl peptidase 4 inhibitor • Sulfonylureas • Biguanides

KEY POINTS

- Most patients with diabetes mellitus take antidiabetic oral and noninsulin injectable medications.
- Hospitalized patients with diabetes mellitus need to be evaluated on admission to determine whether the home diabetes medication regimen can be continued.
- Many of the antidiabetic oral and noninsulin injectable medications need to be discontinued in the hospitalized patient.

INTRODUCTION

Over the past few decades, diabetes mellitus has become a growing epidemic that affects millions of people worldwide each year.[1] The most common treatment plan for patients with type 2 diabetes mellitus (T2DM) includes diet, exercise, and noninsulin antidiabetic medications. Of the 25.8 million people in the United States with diabetes, 58% use only noninsulin antidiabetic medications, and 14% take both insulin and noninsulin antidiabetic medications, which means 72% of patients with diabetes use noninsulin antidiabetic medications.[2] Even if patients are well controlled at home, it is important to evaluate the safety and effectiveness of their home plan they become hospitalized. Many factors during hospitalization may affect the safety and effectiveness of the home plan, including changes in nutrition status (nothing by mouth, tube feeding, and total parental

Disclosure: The author has no relationship with a commercial company that has a direct financial interest in the subject matter or materials discussed in the article, or with a company making a competing product.

The University of Texas at MD Anderson Cancer Center, 1515 Holcombe Boulevard, Houston, TX 77030, USA

* 3306 Southmere Lane, Pearland, TX 77584.

E-mail address: casiska@mdanderson.org

Crit Care Nurs Clin N Am 25 (2013) 39–53

http://dx.doi.org/10.1016/j.ccell.2012.11.012

nutrition), planned and unplanned procedures or surgery, infection, nondiabetes medications that affect blood glucose such as steroids, changes in physical activity, and complications such as renal, hepatic, or heart failure. This article discusses the different classes of noninsulin antidiabetic medications, the mechanism of action, metabolism, elimination, dose form, usual and maximum doses, contraindications, precautions, common adverse reactions, and implications for use in the hospitalized patient.

CLASSES OF ORAL DIABETES MEDICATIONS

There are currently 9 different classes of antidiabetic oral and noninsulin injectable medications on the United States market, which include sulfonylureas (SU), meglitinides (MG), thiazolinediones (TZD), biguanides, α-glucosidase inhibitors (AGI), dipeptidyl peptidase-4 inhibitors (DPP-4), dopamine agonists (DA), glucagon-like peptide-1 analogues (GLP-1), and amylin analogues. Many patients with diabetes mellitus take a combination of noninsulin antidiabetic medications. Each class serves a different role, and affects insulin receptors and glucose production in different ways (Appendix A).

Sulfonylureas

Sulfonylureas were the first oral medications used to manage T2DM, and are one of the most common types of oral hypoglycemic agents used in clinical practice.[3] Sulfonylureas bind to an adenosine triphosphate (ATP)-dependent K^+ channel of the cell membrane of the pancreatic β cell causing release of insulin, enhancing insulin receptor sensitivity, and limiting hepatic glucose production.[4] Sulfonylurea causes the closure of ATP-sensitive potassium channels.[3] The most commonly used sulfonylureas on the United States market include glipizide (Glucotrol, Glucotrol XL), glimepiride (Amaryl), glyburide (Diabeta, Micronase), and micronized glyburide (Glynase).

Glipizide is rapidly absorbed after oral administration, and has an elimination half-life of 2 to 5 hours.[3] It is metabolized in the liver via CYP450 2C9 substrate, and is eliminated 80% in urine and 10% in feces. Glipizide is available in 5-mg and 10-mg scored tablets. Glipizide XL comes in 2.5-mg, 5-mg, and 10-mg extended-release tablets. The usual starting dose is 5 mg daily and the maximum recommended daily dose is 20 mg. If the creatinine clearance is less than 50 mL/min, the dose is decreased by 50%. Contraindications include hypersensitivity to glipizide or the drug class, near-term pregnancy, Type 1 diabetes mellitus (T1DM), and diabetic ketoacidosis (DKA). Precautions include allergy to sulfonamides, renal impairment, hepatic impairment, elderly age, adrenal insufficiency, malnutrition, and glucose 6-phosphate dehydrogenase (G6PD) deficiency. Common adverse reactions include hypoglycemia, weight gain, diarrhea, nausea, rash, pruritus, headache, tremor, nervousness, drowsiness, and photosensitivity. Because of the high risk for causing hypoglycemia, this drug should be discontinued in the hospitalized patient if the patient has decreased food intake, is malnourished, has renal failure, or has a contraindication.

Glimepiride is administered orally and is 99.5% protein bound. It has a half-life of 5 hours initially but increases to 9 hours after multiple dosing. Two metabolites are formed, the cyclohexyl hydroxy methyl derivative and the carboxyl derivative. Glimepiride is metabolized via P450 2C9, and is eliminated 60% in urine and 40% in feces. It is available in 1-mg, 2-mg, and 4-mg tablets, with a usual starting dose of 1 to 2 mg and a maximum daily dose of 8 mg.[3] If the patient has renal impairment, the initial dose should be 1 mg by mouth daily, which should be increased slowly. Contraindications include hypersensitivity to glimepiride or the drug class, T1DM, and DKA. Precautions include allergy to sulfonylamides, renal impairment, hepatic impairment, elderly age, adrenal insufficiency, malnutrition, autonomic neuropathy, and G6PD deficiency. Common adverse reactions include hypoglycemia, weight gain, dizziness, asthenia, nausea, headache, and photosensitivity. Because of the high risk for causing hypoglycemia, this drug should be discontinued in the hospitalized patient if the patient has decreased food intake, is malnourished, has renal failure, or has a contraindication.

Glyburide is administered orally and is highly protein bound via nonionic binding. Its half-life is 10 hours, with 18 to 24 hours' duration in patients with normal renal function. It is metabolized completely in the liver via CYP450 2C9 substrate to 2 metabolites, which are only weakly active. Both the drug and its metabolites are eliminated equally in the urine and feces. The dosage forms comprise 1.25-mg, 2.5-mg, and 5-mg tablets. The usual starting dose is 2.5 to 5 mg daily with a maximum dose of 20 mg. The micronized formulation (Glynase) is not bioequivalent to conventional glyburide (Diabeta, Micronase). Glynase is absorbed within 1 hour with a peak serum concentration after 2 to 3 hours. It comes in 1.5-mg, 3-mg, and 6-mg scored tablets. The usual starting dose is 0.75 to 3 mg daily with a maximum dose of 12 mg daily. Glyburide should not be used in patients with a creatinine clearance of less than 50 mL/min. Contraindications include hypersensitivity to the drug class or glimepiride, near-term pregnancy, creatinine clearance less than 50 mL/min, T1DM, and DKA. Precautions include allergy to sulfonylamides, renal impairment, hepatic impairment, elderly age, adrenal insufficiency, malnutrition, autonomic neuropathy, and G6PD deficiency. Common adverse reactions include hypoglycemia, weight gain, nausea, epigastric discomfort, dyspepsia, blurred vision, drowsiness, elevation of alanine aminotransferase (ALT) and/or aspartate aminotransferase level, rash, and photosensitivity. Because of the high risk for causing hypoglycemia, this drug should be discontinued in the hospitalized patient if the patient has decreased food intake, is malnourished, has renal failure, or has a contraindication.

Meglitinides

Meglitinides are nonsulfonylurea agents that increase insulin secretion by binding to and closing the ATP-sensitive potassium channels.[3] The blockade of potassium channels depolarizes the β cells, which leads to opening of calcium channels and results in the influx of calcium, inducing insulin secretion. There are 2 meglitinides on the United States market, repaglinide (Prandin) and nateglinide (Starlix).

Repaglinide is orally administered, and is a carbamoylmethylbenzoic acid derivative that is rapidly absorbed into the body and eliminated within hours. Its half-life is 1 to 1.4 hours. Because of the rapid absorption and elimination of the agent, repaglinides should be taken with meals. It is metabolized by the liver via CYP450 2C8 3A4 substrate. It is excreted 90% in feces and 8% in urine. Repaglinide is available in 0.5-mg, 1-mg, and 2-mg tablets. The usual starting dose is 0.5 mg with each meal, with a maximum daily dose is 16 mg.[3] If the creatinine clearance is 20 to 40 mL/min, the initial dose is 0.5 mg with each meal, titrating the dose with caution. Use in patients with a creatinine clearance of less than 20 mL/min has not been studied. Contraindications include hypersensitivity to repaglinide or its drug class, T1DM, and DKA. Precautions include severe renal impairment, hepatic impairment, and use with insulin. Common adverse reactions include hypoglycemia, upper respiratory infection, headache, arthralgia, diarrhea, back pain, nausea, vomiting, constipation, dyspepsia, paresthesia, and chest pain. Compared with the sulfonylureas, repaglinide has a lower risk of causing hypoglycemia. This drug should be discontinued in the hospitalized patient if the patient has decreased food intake, is malnourished, has renal failure, or has a contraindication.

Nateglinide is orally administered, and is a D-phenylalanine derivative that binds to potassium channels more quickly than repaglinide. Nateglinide causes a quick and short insulin response that mirrors an after-meal insulin release.[3] Its half-life is 1.5 hours. It is metabolized by the liver via CYP450 2C9 3A4 substrate. Nateglinide is excreted 83% in urine and 10% in feces. It is available in 60-mg and 120-mg tablets. The usual starting dose is 120 mg with each meal, with a maximum recommended daily dose of 360 mg. No adjustment is needed for renal disease. Contraindications include hypersensitivity to nateglinide or its drug class, T1DM, and DKA. Precautions include severe renal impairment, elderly age, malnutrition, adrenal insufficiency, autonomic neuropathy, and hepatic impairment. Common adverse reactions include hypoglycemia, upper respiratory infection, influenza-like symptoms, dizziness, arthropathy, accidental injury, bronchitis, cough, diarrhea, and back pain. Compared with the sulfonylureas, nateglinide has a lower risk of causing hypoglycemia. This drug should be discontinued in the hospitalized patient if the patient has decreased food intake, is malnourished, has renal failure, or has a contraindication.

Thiazolidinediones

Thiazolidinediones are insulin-sensitizing agents that improve the target cell (skeletal muscle, adipose, and liver) response and decrease hepatic gluconeogenesis.[5] This class of diabetes oral agents stimulates a nuclear receptor called peroxisome proliferator–activated receptor γ, which regulates the transcription of several insulin-responsive genes. Studies have shown a correlation between thiazolidinediones and lower blood pressure and cholesterol levels,[6] and these agents have been shown to reduce inflammation and restore vasodilatory effects of insulin in the smooth muscle of the body's vasculature.[7] Thiazoladinediones carry a black-box warning that they may cause or exacerbate congestive heart failure (CHF). It is recommended that patients be observed closely after initiation and after each dose increase for excessive, rapid weight gain, dyspnea, and/or edema, and that discontinuation should be considered if the patient has symptoms of CHF, and is contraindicated in patients with New York Heart Association (NYHA) Class III to IV heart failure. Studies have linked thiazoladinediones to certain positive anticancer characteristics, including arrest of cell growth, induction of apoptosis, and inhibition of cell invasion; for example, thiazoladinediones have been shown to inhibit invasion of pancreatic cancer cells and to block cell-cycle progression.[8] Further studies are being explored to decide whether key particles or molecules associated with thiazoladinediones are also involved in inhibiting cancer growth. The 2 types of thiazoladinediones used in the United States are pioglitazone (Actos) and rosiglitazone (Avandia).

Pioglitazone is orally administered and is highly protein bound. Serum steady state is achieved within 7 days. The half-life is 3 to 7 hours, and the half-life of the metabolites is 16 to 24 hours. Pioglitazone is metabolized by the liver via CYP450 2CB and 3A4 substrate. It is excreted 15% to 30% in urine, with the remainder being excreted through bile and feces. It is available in 15-mg, 30-mg, and 45-mg tablets. The starting dose is 15 to 30 mg daily, with a maximum dose of 45 mg daily. No renal dosage adjustment is needed. Pioglitazone should not be used if the ALT level is greater than 2.5 times the upper limit of normal. Contraindications include hypersensitivity to pioglitazone or its drug class, T1DM, DKA, baseline ALT greater than 2.5 times the upper limit of normal, active bladder cancer, CHF NYHA Class III to IV, and symptoms of CHF. Precautions include CHF NYHA Class I to II, CHF risk, edema, hepatic impairment, history of bladder cancer, use with insulin, and use in female patients (may induce ovulation). Pioglitazone is safe during hospitalization as long as the patient is eating well. Thiazolidinediones are not effective in the acute management of hyperglycemia because it takes approximately 6 weeks to reach a steady state.

Rosiglitazone is orally administered, rapidly absorbed, and highly protein bound (99.8%). Its half-life is 3 to 4 hours, and it is highly metabolized by the liver CYP450 2C8 2C9 substrate. Excretion is 64% in urine and 23% in feces. Rosiglitazone is available in 2-mg, 4-mg, and 8-mg tablets. The usual starting dose is 4 mg (administered as 4 mg once a day or 2 mg twice a day). The recommended maximum daily dose is 8 mg. No dosage adjustment is needed for renal disease. At present, rosiglitazone has restricted distribution in the United States. The prescriber must justify and gain permission from the Food and Drug Administration before prescribing. Contraindications include hypersensitivity to pioglitazone or its drug class, T1DM, DKA, baseline ALT greater than 2.5 times the upper limit of normal, active bladder cancer, CHF NYHA Class III to IV, symptoms of CHF, and acute coronary syndrome. Precautions include CHF NYHA Class I to II, CHF risk, edema, hepatic impairment, use with a sulfonylurea, use with insulin, and use in female patients (may induce ovulation). Rosiglitazone is generally safe in the hospitalized patient who does not have contraindications or at high risk for CHF or liver failure. Thiazolidinediones are not effective in the acute management of hyperglycemia because it takes approximately 6 weeks to reach a steady state.

Biguanides

Biguanides are one of the most commonly used classes of diabetes oral agent. This class decreases hepatic glucose production and gastrointestinal (GI) glucose absorption, and increases insulin sensitivity of specific target cells.[9] Insulin secretion is unchanged, so it does not cause hypoglycemia; it has an antihyperglycemic action rather than a hypoglycemic action. Other benefits include a decrease in fatty acid oxidation by 10% to 20% and a slight increase in glucose oxidation. The biguanide class is often used in combination with other classes of diabetes oral agents. The biguanide class has only one drug in its class, which is metformin (Glucophage, Glucophage XR, Fortamet, Glumetza, and Riomet).

Metformin is administered orally as immediate-release tablets, a solution, or extended-release tablets. It is distributed rapidly into peripheral body tissues and fluids, and appears to distribute slowly into the erythrocytes and slowly into GI tissues. Its half-life is 6.2 hours in plasma and 17.6 hours in the blood. The liver does not metabolize metformin. It is excreted largely unchanged by the kidneys through an active tubular process. A small percentage is excreted in the feces. Metformin is available in 500-mg, 850-mg, and 1000-mg immediate-release tablets, and in 500-mg and 750-mg extended-release tablets. The usual starting dose for immediate release is 500 mg twice daily or 850 mg daily. The maximum recommended daily dose is 2550 mg. The starting dose for the extended-release form is 500 mg every evening, titrating the dose by 500 mg per week to a maximum of 2000 mg daily. There is no dosage reduction for poor renal function because metformin is contraindicated for elevated creatinine clearance above 1.4 mL/min in women and 1.5 mL/min in men.[9] Contraindications include allergy to metformin, elevated creatinine clearance above 1.4 mL/min in women and 1.5 mL/min in men, metabolic acidosis, lactic acidosis, iodinated contrast, hypoxemia, dehydration, sepsis, surgery, and hepatic disease. Precautions include CHF, elderly age, alcohol abuse, and patients at high risk for hypoglycemia. Common reactions include diarrhea, nausea, vomiting, flatulence, asthenia, indigestion, abdominal discomfort, anorexia, headache, metallic taste, rash, and induction of ovulation. When patients are hospitalized, metformin is usually discontinued because of safety issues. If it is continued, it will need to be temporarily held approximately 48 hours before and after surgery, imaging procedures with iodinated contrast, or concomitant use of nephrotoxic medications. Metformin may be resumed once the renal function is documented as normal.

α-Glucosidase Inhibitors

α-Glucosidase inhibitors prevent the GI enzymes maltase and sucrose from being absorbed in the lining of the gut, decreasing postprandial hyperglycemia.[10] Common side effects include abdominal discomfort such as bloating, diarrhea, and flatulence. α-Glucosidase inhibitors do not pose the same adverse side effects as sulfonylureas, such as weight gain and hypoglycemia.[10] If a patient is taking α-glucosidase inhibitors in conjunction with sulfonylureas and hypoglycemia occurs, the best treatment option is for the patient to take an oral dextrose supplement rather than a sucrose supplement. Two oral α-glucosidase inhibitors are available on the United States market: acarbose (Precose) and miglitol (Glyset).

Acarbose is administered orally and has low systemic absorption. The mechanism of action occurs locally in the GI tract. It is metabolized within the GI tract via intestinal microbial flora, intestinal hydrolysis, and the activity of digestive enzymes. The excretion is 51% in feces and 34% in urine. Acarbose is available in 25-mg, 50-mg, and 100-mg tablets. The usual starting dose is 25 mg with each meal, with a maximum dose of 100 mg with each meal. There is no dosage reduction for renal disease; however, it is contraindicated if the creatinine clearance is greater than 2 mL/min. Contraindications include hypersensitivity to acarbose or its drug class, DKA, cirrhosis, inflammatory bowel disease, colonic ulceration, partial GI obstruction, risk of GI obstruction, malabsorption syndromes, and a creatinine clearance greater than 2 mL/min. Precautions include renal impairment. Common adverse reactions include flatulence, diarrhea, abdominal pain, and elevated liver function tests. Acarbose is infrequently used in the hospitalized patient because of the propensity for the patient to miss meals.

Miglitol is administered orally and is distributed primarily into extracellular fluid, and is minimally protein bound. Unlike acarbose, miglitol is not metabolized in any way. It is excreted unchanged by the kidneys. The half-life is 2 hours. Miglitol is available in 25-mg, 50-mg, and 100-mg tablets. The usual starting dose is 25 mg with each meal, and the maximum dose is 100 mg with each meal. There is no dosage reduction for renal disease; however, it is contraindicated if the creatinine clearance is greater than 2 mL/min. Contraindications include hypersensitivity to miglitol or its drug class, DKA, inflammatory bowel disease, colonic ulceration, partial GI obstruction, and creatinine clearance greater than 2 mL/min. Precautions include renal impairment. Common adverse reactions include flatulence, diarrhea, abdominal pain, and rash. Miglitol is infrequently used in the hospitalized patient because of the propensity for the patient to miss meals.

Dipeptidyl Peptidase-4 Inhibitors

Dipeptidyl peptidase-4 (DPP-4) inhibitors increase and lengthen the incretin hormone, which originates from the intestinal tract and stimulates the release of insulin from the pancreas in a glucose-dependent manner.[11] In addition to affecting incretin hormone release, DDP-4 inhibitors also improve serum glucose control without posing the risk of hypoglycemia or weight gain. There are 3 DPP-4 inhibitors on the United States market: linagliptin (Tradjenta), saxagliptin (Onglyza), and sitagliptin (Januvia).

Linagliptin is administered orally and is extensively distributed in the tissues. The half-life is 12 hours. The drug is minimally metabolized and it is a weak to moderate inhibitor of CYP3A4, but does not inhibit other CYP isozymes and is not an inducer of CYP isozymes. It is excreted 80% in feces and 5% in urine, and is available in 5-mg tablets. There is only one dose for each patient, which is 5 mg, and there is no adjustment for renal impairment. Contraindications include hypersensitivity to linagliptin and its drug class, T1DM, and DKA. Common adverse reactions include nasopharyngitis, hypoglycemia, and hyperuricemia. Linagliptin has few side effects, does not cause hypoglycemia, and can be given without regard to meals; however, it may not manage acute hyperglycemia in hospitalized patients.

Saxagliptin is administered orally. Its half-life is 2.5 hours. Metabolized by the liver extensively, it is a p-glycoprotein substrate and a cytochrome P450 3A4/5 enzyme system substrate. It is excreted 75% in urine and 22% in feces. Saxagliptin is available in 2.5-mg and 5-mg tablets. For patients with normal renal function, the dose is 5 mg daily. If the creatinine clearance is less than 50 mL/min, the dose is 2.5 mg daily. If the patient is on hemodialysis, the dose is given after dialysis.[11] Contraindications include hypersensitivity to saxagliptin and its drug class, T1DM, and DKA. Precautions include renal impairment. Common adverse reactions include upper respiratory infection, urinary tract infection, headache, hypoglycemia, vomiting, peripheral edema, abdominal pain, gastroenteritis, and hypersensitivity reaction. Saxagliptin has few side effects, does not cause hypoglycemia, and can be given without regard to meals; however, it may not manage acute hyperglycemia in hospitalized patients.

Sitagliptin is administered orally and is not highly bound to plasma proteins. It is minimally metabolized by the liver via CYP450 2C8 3A4 substrate. Its half-life is 12.4 hours. It is excreted 87% in urine and 13% in feces. Sitagliptin is available in 25-mg, 50-mg, and 100-mg tablets. The usual starting dose is 100 mg daily. If the creatinine clearance is between 30 and 49 mL/min, the dose is reduced to 50 mg daily. If the creatinine clearance is less than 30 mL/min, the dose is reduced to 25 mg daily. Contraindications include hypersensitivity to sitagliptin and its drug class, T1DM, and DKA. Precautions include renal impairment and history of pancreatitis. Common adverse reactions include upper respiratory infection, headache, diarrhea, abdominal pain, and arthralgia. Sitagliptin has few side effects, does not cause hypoglycemia, and can be given without regard to meals; however, it may not manage acute hyperglycemia in hospitalized patients.

Dopamine Agonists

Bromocriptine mesylate (Cycloset) is a dopamine agonist that was previously used to treat prolactinemia and Parkinson disease; however, it recently received an indication to treat T2DM. Its mechanism of action is not well understood but is thought to lower glucose by a central signaling phenomenon. It stimulates dopamine receptors, inhibits anterior pituitary prolactin secretion, and modulates neurotransmitters centrally. Bromocriptine lowers glucose without increasing insulin levels, and is the only one medication in this class.

Bromocriptine is administered orally and binds extensively to serum albumin, and does not distribute into erythrocytes. Its half-life is biphasic, at 4 to 4.5 hours and 15 hours. It is metabolized by the liver via CYP450 3A4 substrate. It is excreted 95% in bile and 2.5% to 5.5% in urine. Bromocriptine is available in 0.8-mg tablets.

The starting dose is 0.8 mg daily and the maximum dose is 4.8 mg daily. There are no recommendations for reducing the dose for impaired renal function. Contraindications include hypersensitivity to bromocriptine, its drug class and ergot derivatives, T1DM, DKA, migraine with syncope, and breastfeeding. Precautions include renal impairment, hepatic impairment, use with concurrent antihypertensives, and psychosis. Common adverse reactions include nausea, asthenia, headache, rhinitis, sinusitis, dizziness, constipation, influenza syndrome, diarrhea, amblyopia, dyspepsia, somnolence, vomiting, infection, anorexia, hypoglycemia, and orthostatic hypotension. Bromocriptine is not recommended for use in hospitalized patients, because the mechanism of action is not well understood and because there are few data concerning the safety of use in hospitalized patients.

Incretine Mimetics

Glucagon-like peptide-1 (GLP-1) enhances insulin secretion after release from the gut into the systemic circulation. Incretine mimetics enhance glucose-dependent insulin secretion and other antihyperglycemic actions of incretions, and also suppress glucagon secretion, slow gastric emptying, and induce central appetite suppression. The effects are dependent on the serum glucose level and will not occur if the blood glucose is less than 65 mg/dL. There are 3 incretin mimetics on the United States market: exenatide (Byetta), exenatide extended-release (Bydureon), and liraglutide (Victoza).

Exenatide is administered subcutaneously. Its half-life is 2.4 hours and it is minimally metabolized. Exenatide is excreted predominately by glomerular filtration with subsequent proteolytic degradation. It is available in a 5-µg per dose pen and a 10-µg per dose pen. The starting dose is 5 µg twice daily with the 2 largest meals, and the maximum dose is 10 µg twice daily with the 2 largest meals. There is no reduced dose with mild renal impairment. It is contraindicated if the creatinine clearance is less than 30 mL/min. Contraindications include hypersensitivity to exenatide and its drug class, T1DM, DKA, severe GI disease, history of pancreatitis, and creatinine clearance less than 30 mL/min. Precautions include creatinine clearance of 30 to 50 mL/min, renal transplant, concurrent use of nephrotoxic medications, and concurrent medications requiring rapid onset. Common adverse reactions include nausea, vomiting, diarrhea, hypoglycemia, constipation, headache, and dyspepsia. There is limited experience with use of exenatide in hospitalized patients. Exenatide needs to be given in relation to a meal, which may be difficult in hospitalized patients. It may delay absorption of medications, decrease appetite, and contribute to nausea and vomiting.

Exenatide extended-release is a once-weekly subcutaneous injection of exenatide. The metabolism and excretion are the same as for exenatide. It is available in a 2-mg kit. The dosing is 2 mg subcutaneously per week. Exenatide extended-release carries a black-box warning concerning an increased risk for thyroid c-cell tumor. Contraindications include a history of medullary thyroid cancer, current medullary thyroid cancer, a family history of medullary thyroid cancer, multiple endocrine neoplasia syndrome type 2, intramuscular or intravenous administration, hypersensitivity to exenatide and its drug class, T1DM, DKA, severe GI disease, history of pancreatitis, and creatinine clearance less than 30 mL/min. Precautions include creatinine clearance 30 to 50 mL/min, renal transplant, concurrent use of nephrotoxic medications, and concurrent medications requiring rapid onset. Common adverse reactions include nausea, vomiting, diarrhea, hypoglycemia, constipation, headache, injection-site reaction, and dyspepsia. Exenetide extended-release has not been used widely in hospitalized patients. It may delay absorption of medications and decrease appetite, and contribute to nausea and vomiting.

Loraglutide is administered subcutaneously and is more than 98% bound to plasma protein. The half-life is 13 hours. It is minimally metabolized via CYP450. It is excreted 6% in urine and 5% in feces. Loraglutide is available in a prefilled pen containing 18 mg/3 mL. The pen delivers 0.6 μg, 1.2 μg, or 1.8 μg per injection. The starting dose is 0.6 μg daily and maximum 1.8 μg daily. There is no dosage adjustment for renal impairment. It carries a black-box warning concerning an increased risk for thyroid c-cell tumor. Contraindications include a history of medullary thyroid cancer, current medullary thyroid cancer, a family history of medullary thyroid cancer, multiple endocrine neoplasia syndrome type 2, hypersensitivity to exenatide and its drug class, T1DM, and DKA. Precautions include gastroparesis, concurrent use with oral medications requiring rapid onset, and history of pancreatitis. Common adverse reactions include nausea, vomiting, diarrhea, constipation, headache, injection-site reaction, anorexia, decreased appetite, upper respiratory infection influenza, urinary tract infection, dizziness, sinusitis, nasopharyngitis, fatigue, back pain, hypertension, and dyspepsia. Loraglutide has not been used widely in hospitalized patients. It may delay absorption of medications and decrease appetite, and contribute to nausea and vomiting.

Amylin Agonists

Amylin is produced by β cells and is cosecreted with insulin, and works in concert with insulin to regulate postprandial glucose concentrations. Amylin affects glucose concentrations by slowing of gastric emptying without altering the overall absorption of nutrients, by suppression of postprandial glucagon secretion, and by centrally mediated modulation of appetite leading to decreased caloric intake. There is only one amylin agonist on the United States market, pramlintide (Symlin).

Pramlintide is administered by subcutaneous injection. It is not extensively bound to blood cells or albumin; approximately 40% of the drug is bound in plasma. The half-life is approximately 48 minutes with the therapeutic effects lasting approximately 3 hours. It is extensively metabolized by the kidney. Pramlintide comes in 3 forms: Symlin vial (0.6 mg/mL), Symlin Pen 120 (1000 μg/mL), and Symlin Pen 60 (1000 μg/mL). The starting dose for patients with T1DM is 15 μg with each meal, with a target dose of 60 μg with each meal. The starting dose for T2DM is 60 μg with each meal, with a maximum dose of 120 μg with each meal. No dose adjustment is needed in those with a creatinine clearance greater than 20 mL/min. Contraindications include hypersensitivity to pramlintide or its drug class, hypersensitivity to cresol, gastroparesis, and hypoglycemia unawareness or history of severe hypoglycemia. Precautions include breastfeeding, children, dialysis, diarrhea, driving or operating machinery, fever, elderly age, infection, osteoporosis, pregnancy, renal failure, surgery, thyroid disease, tobacco smoking, trauma, and vomiting. Common adverse reactions include abdominal pain, anorexia, arthralgia, blurred vision, coma, confusion, diaphoresis, dizziness, fatigue, headache, hypoglycemia, injection-site reaction, irritability, lipodystrophy, nausea, pallor, palpitations, pharyngitis, pruritus, sinus tachycardia, and vomiting. Pramlintide may be used in hospitalized patients who are eating well and are receiving prandial insulin.

SUMMARY

Diabetes mellitus is a growing epidemic that affects millions of Americans each year. Health care providers should be aware of the different classes of diabetes oral agents prescribed to patients, and the risks and benefits associated with each type of medication. With the increase in cases of T2DM, the use of oral hypoglycemic agents is increasing concomitantly, providing ongoing opportunities to raise awareness about theses agents' adverse side effects such as cardiovascular risks and renal failure.

REFERENCES

1. Polikandrioti M, Dokoutsidou H. The role of exercise and nutrition in type II diabetes mellitus management. Health Sci J 2009;3:216–21.
2. National Diabetes Information Clearinghouse (NDIC). National diabetes statistics, 2011. Available at: http://diabetes.niddk.nih.gov/dm/pubs/statistics/#Treatment. Accessed August 26, 2012.
3. Rendell M. The role of sulphonylureas in the management of type 2 diabetes mellitus. Drugs 2004;64(12):1339–58.
4. Lu FR, Shen L, Qin Y, et al. Clinical observation on *Trigonella foenum-graecum* L. Total saponins in combination with sulfonylureas in the treatment of type 2 diabetes mellitus. Chin J Integr Med 2008;14:56–60.
5. Krentz A, Friedmann P. Type 2 diabetes, psoriasis and thiazolidinediones. Int J Clin Pract 2006;60:362–3.
6. Sarafidis P, Bakris G. Protection of the kidney by thiazolidinediones: an assessment from bench to bedside. Kidney Int 2006;70:1223–33.
7. Granberry M, Hawkins J, Franks A. Thiazolidinediones in patients with type 2 diabetes mellitus and heart failure. Am J Health Syst Pharm 2007;64:931–6.
8. Okumura T. Mechanisms by which thiazolidinediones induce anti-cancer effects in cancers in digestive organs. J Gastroenterol 2010;45:1097–102.
9. Chwieduk CM. Sitagliptin/metformin fixed-dose combination in patients with type 2 diabetes mellitus. Drugs 2011;71:349–61.
10. Patil S, Ghadyale V, Taklikar S, et al. Insulin secretagogue, alpha-glucosidase and antioxidant activity of some selected spices in streptozotocin-induced diabetic rats. Plant Foods Hum Nutr 2011;66:85–90. http://dx.doi.org/10.1007/s11130-011-0215-7.
11. Neumiller J, Campbell R. Saxagliptin: a dipeptidyl peptidase-4 inhibitor for the treatment of type 2 diabetes mellitus. Am J Health Syst Pharm 2010;67:1515–25.

APPENDIX A: ORAL AND INJECTABLE NONINSULIN ANTIDIABETIC MEDICATIONS

Medication Class Generic (Trademark)	Risk for Hypoglycemia Common Adverse Effects	Precautions	Contraindications	Renal Dosing	Implications for the Hospitalized Patient
Sulfonylureas:					
Glimepiride (Amaryl), Glipizide (Glucotrol, Glucotrol XL) Glyburide (Diabeta, Glynase PresTab, Micronase)	Yes Hypoglycemia, weight gain	Impaired renal and hepatic function, adrenal or pituitary insufficiency, elderly age, malnourished	DKA, T1DM, allergy	Glipizide: reduce dose by 50%. Glimepiride: start with 1 mg daily Glyburide: do not use if CrCl is <50 mL/min	Because of the high risk for causing hypoglycemia, this class should be discontinued in the hospitalized patient if the patient has decreased food intake, is malnourished, has renal failure, or has a contraindication
Meglitinides:					
Nateglinide (Starlix) Repaglinide (Prandin)	Yes Hypoglycemia (less risk compared with sulfonylureas)	Renal insufficiency, liver disease, use with insulin, adrenal insufficiency, surgery, trauma, elderly age, pituitary insufficiency, malnourished	DKA, T1DM, allergy, use with gemfibrozil	Repaglinide: Reduce usual dose by half if CrCl 20–40 mL/min. Not studied in those with CrCl <20 mL/min Nateglinide: No dose adjustment needed	Compared with the sulfonylureas, meglitinides have a lower risk of causing hypoglycemia. This drug class should be discontinued in the hospitalized patient if the patient has decreased food intake, is malnourished, has renal failure, or has a contraindication

(continued on next page)

Medication Class Generic (Trademark)	Risk for Hypoglycemia Common Adverse Effects	Precautions	Contraindications	Renal Dosing	Implications for the Hospitalized Patient
Thiazolidinediones:					
Pioglitazone (Actos) Rosiglitizone (Avandia)	No Increased risk of bladder cancer if used >1 y duration, increased risk of fracture in females, may cause ovulation in females in some premenopausal anovulatory women, weight gain, edema	Elevated ALT, dyspnea, rapid weight gain, use with insulin, use in patients with coronary artery disease	DKA, T1DM, allergy, Class III or IV heart failure, ALT >2.5 times ULM	No dose adjustment needed	Thiazoladinediones are generally safe in the hospitalized patient that does not have contraindications or is high risk for CHF or liver failure. They are not effective in acute management of hyperglycemia because it takes approximately 6 wk to reach steady state
Biguanides:					
Metformin (Glucophage, Glucophage XR, Fortamet, Riomet)	No Nausea, vomiting, diarrhea, flatulence, low serum B12. May cause ovulation in anovulatory and premenopausal PCOS patients	Malnourished, debilitation, infection-induced stress, fever, trauma, elderly	Black-Box Warning: Lactic acidosis is a rare but potentially severe consequence of therapy with metformin. Do not use or discontinue in those with unstable, acute CHF who are at risk of hypoperfusion and hypoxemia, renal dysfunction	Discontinue if the creatinine is >1.5 in men, or >1.4 in women	When patients are hospitalized, metformin is usually discontinued owing to safety issues. If it is continued, it will need to be temporarily be held approximately 48 h before and after surgery, imaging procedures with iodinated contrast or

	Hypoglycemia	Side effects	Precautions/Interactions	Contraindications	Renal dosing	Comments
				(creatinine >1.4 in women and >1.5 in men), dehydration, sepsis, surgery, tests involving the injection of dye, hepatic disease, excessive or chronic alcohol consumption, hypersensitivity, metabolic acidosis, DKA		concomitant use of nephrotoxic medications. Metformin may be resumed once the renal function is documented to be normal
α-Glucosidase inhibitors:						
Acarbose (Precose) Miglitol (Glyset)	No	Abdominal pain, diarrhea, elevated serum transaminases, flatulence	Concurrent use with sulfonylureas. If hypoglycemia occurs, treat with oral dextrose not sucrose	DKA, T1DM, allergy, cirrhosis, inflammatory bowel disease, colonic ulceration, partial intestinal obstruction	Do not use if the creatinine is >2	α-Glucosidase inhibitors are infrequently used in the hospitalized patient because of the propensity for the patient to miss meals
Dipeptidyl peptidase-4 inhibitors:						
Linagliptin (Tradjenta) Saxagliptin (Onglyza) Sitagliptin phosphate (Januvia)	No	Comparable with placebo, abdominal pain, diarrhea, nasopharyngitis, nausea headache, URI	Renal impairment, acute pancreatitis, use with insulin or sulfonylureas	DKA, T1DM, allergy	Linagliptin: no dose adjustment Saxagliptin: 2.5 mg/d if CrCl <50 mL/min Sitagliptin: 50 mg/d if CrCl 30–50 mL/min; 25 mg/d if CrCl <30 mL/min	Has few side effects, does not cause hypoglycemia, and can be given without regard to meals; however, it may not manage acute hyperglycemia in hospitalized patients

(continued on next page)

Medication Class Generic (Trademark)	Risk for Hypoglycemia Common Adverse Effects	Precautions	Contraindications	Renal Dosing	Implications for the Hospitalized Patient
Dopamine agonists:					
Bromocriptine mesylate (Cycloset)	No Nausea, asthenia, headache, rhinitis, sinusitis, dizziness	Syncopal migraine, breastfeeding, renal impairment, hepatic impairment, concurrent antihypertensives, psychosis	DKA, T1DM, allergy	No data available	Bromocriptine is not recommended for use in hospitalized patients because the mechanism of action is not well understood and because there are few data concerning the safety of use in hospitalized patients
Incretin mimetics:					
Exenatide (Byetta) Exenatide extended-release (Bydureon) Liraglutide (Victoza)	No Diarrhea, nausea, vomiting	Risk for pancreatitis, renal failure	DKA, T1DM, allergy, do not use liraglutide or Exenatide extended-release in those with a history or family history of medullary thyroid cancer	Do not use if CrCl <30 mL/min	There is limited experience with use of incretin mimetics in hospitalized patients. Exenatide needs to be given in relation to a meal, which may be difficult in hospitalized patients. It may delay

Amylin agonists:

Drug		Adverse effects		Contraindications	Renal dosing	Notes
Pramlintide (Symlin)	No	Nausea, headache, vomiting, anorexia, severe hypoglycemia (not directly caused by pramlintide but by the combination of insulin with pramlintide)	Patients at high risk of severe hypoglycemia	DKA, allergy, gastroparesis, current prokinetic agent use, hypoglycemia unawareness, HbA1c >9%	No dose adjustment in those with CrCl >20 mL/min; not tested in those with CrCl <20 mL/min	absorption of medications, decrease appetite, and contribute to nausea and vomiting. Pramlintide may be used in hospitalized patients who are eating well and are receiving prandial insulin

Abbreviations: ALT, alanine aminotransferase; CHF, congestive heart failure; CrCl, creatinine clearance; DKA, diabetic ketoacidosis; HbA1c, hemoglobin A1c; PCOS, polycystic ovary syndrome; T1DM, type 1 diabetes mellitus; ULM, upper limit of normal; URI, upper respiratory infection.

Use of Insulin in the Noncritically Ill-hospitalized Patients with Hyperglycemia and Diabetes

Becky Childers, RN, MSNspEd, CDE[a],*,
Celia M. Levesque, RN, MSN, NP-C, CNS-BC, BC-ADM, CDE[b]

KEYWORDS

- Diabetes • Insulin • Diabetes medications • Hyperglycemia

KEY POINTS

- Hyperglycemia is common and often unrecognized among hospitalized patients.
- Hyperglycemia can complicate features of underlying disease and some therapies.
- It is important for the nurse to understand the basics of insulin and its use in the hospitalized patient.

INTRODUCTION

Diabetes is considered to be a public health crisis that affects at least 8.3% of the population in the United States.[1] Furthermore, the Centers for Disease Control and Prevention estimates that 79 million Americans aged 20 years and above have prediabetes.[2] Patients with diabetes have a 2.2 to 4-fold increased incidence of hospitalization compared with the nondiabetes population. More than 7.7 million Americans with diabetes are hospitalized each year. One in every 5 admissions is related to diabetes, and a person with diabetes occupies 12% to 25% of all hospital beds. McDonnell found 38% of all hospitalized patients will have hyperglycemia and one-third of those do not have a history of diabetes.[3] Umpierrez found that hyperglycemia was present in 38% of patients admitted to the hospital as either a primary or secondary diagnosis, of whom 26% had a known history of diabetes and 12% had no history of diabetes before admission. In addition, new hyperglycemic patients had longer hospital stays and a higher admission rate to an intensive care unit and were less likely to be

Disclosure: The author has no relationship with a commercial company that has a direct financial interest in the subject matter or materials discussed in the article or with a company making a competing product.
[a] St Joseph Medical Center, 1401 St Joseph Parkway, 2nd Floor SKS Building, Houston, TX 77002, USA; [b] Department of Endocrine Neoplasia and Hormonal Disorders, The University of Texas MD Anderson Cancer Center, PO Box 301402, Unit 1461, Houston, TX 77230-1402, USA
* Corresponding author.
E-mail address: becky.childers@sjmctx.com

Crit Care Nurs Clin N Am 25 (2013) 55–70
http://dx.doi.org/10.1016/j.ccell.2012.11.002
0899-5885/13/$ – see front matter © 2013 Elsevier Inc. All rights reserved.

discharged to home, frequently requiring transfer to a transitional care unit or nursing home facility. See **Fig. 1** for the average length of stay for patients with normoglycemia, known diabetes, and those with new hyperglycemia. The results indicated that in-hospital hyperglycemia is a common finding and represents an important marker of poor clinical outcome and mortality in patients with and without a history of diabetes.[4] Olson and colleagues discussed the many factors that contribute to the development of hyperglycemia in hospitalized patients without diabetes and poor control in those with diabetes. They found that hyperglycemia is common and often unrecognized among hospitalized patients and is an indicator of poor outcome, increased length of stay, and cost.[5] Hyperglycemia can complicate features of underlying disease and some therapies. However, extreme manifestation of glucose can be prevented or controlled through the application of evidence–based guidelines and sound medical practice for inpatient glycemic control, with proper use of insulin through the use of assessment and identification of hyperglycemia, routine serum glucose measurement, and proper insulin administration. This article discusses physiology and types of diabetes, glycemic targets in the noncritical care setting, factors that contribute to hyperglycemia and hypoglycemia in the hospitalized patient, insulin types, common insulin regimens used in the hospital setting, and implications for the nurse.

PHYSIOLOGY AND TYPES OF DIABETES

Glucose homeostasis involves many factors including insulin secretion, peripheral insulin use, production of endogenous glucose, and consumption of oral nutrition. The pancreas automatically releases insulin to move glucose from the bloodstream into the cells. This process does not occur properly if insulin is not present. Diabetes is a metabolic disorder occurring when the patient has a relative or absolute insulin deficiency resulting in hyperglycemia.[6] Common types of diabetes include Type 1 (T1DM), Type 2 (T2DM), pregestational, and gestational diabetes. Type 1 diabetes mellitus is an autoimmune disease secondary to a T-cell–mediated destruction of the beta cell that leads to beta cell destruction and absolute insulin deficiency. A patient with T1DM requires daily exogenous insulin to sustain life. Omission of insulin can quickly lead to diabetic ketoacidosis (DKA). Patients with T2DM have hyperglycemia due to relative insulin deficiency secondary to insulin resistance. The treatment of T2DM ranges from diet controlled only to a combination of oral agents and insulin. Patients with T2DM are at a lower risk for the development of DKA compared with those with T1DM; however, DKA can occur in patients with T2DM. Diabetes is a chronic disease that requires individualized treatment to prevent severe glucose excursions while hospitalized.

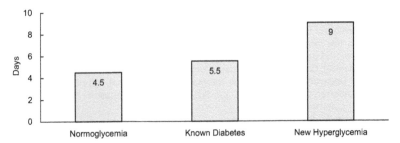

Fig. 1. Average length of stay for hospitalized patients with normoglycemia, known diabetes, and those with new hyperglycemia.

GLYCEMIC TARGETS IN THE NONCRITICAL CARE SETTING

The goal for glucose control in hospitalized patients is to avoid the undesirable short-term effects of hypoglycemia and hyperglycemia by regulating the blood glucose. The American Diabetes Association recommends a preprandial blood glucose level of less than 140 mg/dL and a random blood glucose level of less than 180 mg/dL.[7] The Endocrine Society also recommends a premeal blood glucose level of less than 140 mg/dL and a random blood glucose level of less than 180 mg/dL, with the caveat that targets modified according to clinical status.[8] A lower target may be set for a patient who is not at high risk for hypoglycemia and can safely achieve a lower target. A higher target may be set for those who have a history of severe hypoglycemia unawareness and a limited life expectancy or who are unable to communicate. Kitabchi and colleagues examined the results of randomized clinical trials of strict inpatients glycemic control in medical and surgical intensive care units and recommend a preprandial blood glucose level of 100 to 130 mg/dL and a random blood glucose level of less than 180 mg/dL. They also stressed the importance of avoiding hypoglycemia, especially in critically ill patients who may not be able to communicate. Critically ill patients may have factors that compromise the accuracy of the bedside glucose meter, such as low hematocrit level, hypoxia, or the use of interfering medications such as dopamine. Hypoglycemia with blood glucose levels of less than 40 mg/dL is associated with the near doubling of mortality compared with those with no hypoglycemia.[9]

FACTORS CONTRIBUTING TO HYPERGLYCEMIA IN HOSPITALIZED PATIENTS

Many factors contribute to the development of hyperglycemia in the hospitalized patient. The stress response occurs commonly in patients who are acutely ill, have surgery, sepsis, stroke, burns, trauma, neoplasia etc. In patients without a history of hyperglycemia, physiologic stress can increase the levels of endogenous counter-regulatory hormones (cortisol, glucagon, growth hormone, and epinephrine) and increased inflammatory mediators (tumor necrosis factor α, interleukin 1, interleukin 6), which can lead to hyperglycemia. These mediators promote peripheral and hepatic insulin resistance, increased glycogenolysis and gluconeogenesis, and the enhanced peripheral breakdown of substrates. Exogenous causes of hyperglycemia include many medications (especially steroids), total parental nutrition, enteral feedings, and intravenous dextrose. Patients with T2DM have an underlying beta cell failure combined with increased peripheral insulin resistance and when exposed to the same stressors, may develop a deterioration of their usual glycemic control. Patients with T1DM have absolute insulin deficiency and will experience a deterioration of their usual glycemic control unless the insulin regimen is altered to match their needs. Other factors that contribute to hyperglycemia in hospitalized patients includes the use of sliding scale insulin regimens, missed insulin doses, late insulin doses, unpredictable eating, and prolonged nothing by mouth (NPO) status. Conditions such as renal insufficiency, liver disease, and malnutrition may contribute to hypoglycemia (**Table 1**).[10–13]

TYPES OF INSULIN

Insulin is a hormone that is required for normal carbohydrate, protein, and fat metabolism. With the discovery of insulin in 1921, patients with T1DM were able to live a longer and better quality life. Today, technology allows for the production of synthetic human insulin, which has replaced beef and pork insulin in the United States. Insulin analogues

Table 1
The Endocrine Society's recommendations for calculating insulin doses for the noncritically ill hospitalized patient with T2DM

Step 1: Calculate the total daily insulin dose
   0.2–0.3 units per kilogram if older than 69 years, and/or glomerular filtration rate is less than 60 mL/min
   0.4 units per kilogram if not meeting the criteria mentioned earlier and the blood glucose level is 140–200 mg/dL
   0.5 units per kilogram if not meeting the criteria mentioned earlier and the blood glucose is level 201–400 mg/dL

Step 2: Distribute approximately 50% basal and 50% bolus

Step 3: Give the total basal dose as 1 dose per day using glargine insulin or 2 times per day using detemir or NPH insulin

Step 4: Divide the total bolus dose by 3 to calculate the meal dose.

Step 5: Choose a correctional dose:
   Resistant: for patients requiring more than 80 units of insulin per day or are receiving glucocorticoids
   Usual: for those not meeting the criteria for resistant or sensitive
   Sensitive: for those who are elderly, not eating, or have renal impairment

Correctional Insulin Scale			
Blood Glucose mg/dL	Insulin-sensitive	Usual	Insulin-resistant
141–180	2	4	6
181–220	4	6	8
221–260	6	8	10
261–300	8	10	12
301–350	10	12	14
351–400	12	14	16
Over 400	14	16	18

are developed by modifying the amino acid sequence of the insulin molecule, which allows developers to alter the onset, peak, and duration of the analogue.

The types of insulin include rapid-acting, short-acting, intermediate-acting, and long-acting insulin. The rapid and long-acting insulin are all insulin analogues, and the short and intermediate-acting insulin are human insulin. Some insulin brands are premixed, and some insulin types may be mixed in a syringe. Each is categorized by the onset of action, peak, and duration. Onset means the time it takes the insulin to begin having an effect on lowering blood glucose, peak is the time the action of the insulin is most effective, and duration refers to how long it lasts. Understanding the onset, peak, and duration of a type of insulin, given subcutaneously, will help the provider to manage the blood glucose level during hospitalization. The concentration of insulin in the United States is 100 or 500 units per milliliter, with U-100 more commonly used. Insulin is also available in fixed amounts of intermediate-acting insulin with short or rapid-acting insulin (70% neutral protamine Hagedorn [NPH]/30% regular, 50% NPH/50% regular, and 75% NPL/25% insulin lispro).

The onset, peak, and duration of the insulin types have been developed to pattern after the natural expected release of insulin. Basal insulin mimics the low, steady release of insulin for managing the fasting blood sugar level before meals and overnight. Basal insulin NPH has a 1 to 2 hour time to onset of action, peaks between 4 and 8 hours, and duration of 10 to 12 hours. The peak of NPH can place the inpatient at risk with hypoglycemia if NPO or poor nutritional intake and is dosed 2 times daily to provide continuous basal coverage. Insulin detemir/Levemir and glargine/Lantus are given once daily to most patients, with the exception of some patients given detemir/Levemir 2 times a day. These types of insulin have their onset of action in 1 to 2 hours and when dosed once daily have an essentially flat basal insulin profile that is less likely to lead to hypoglycemia when the patient is NPO or limited intake by mouth. An important note is to administer the insulin dose within an hour of the same time each day to have the most benefits of the action and duration of the insulin.

Bolus insulin is needed for meals and correction of hyperglycemia. Bolus insulin is provided as a rapid-acting analogue or as a regular insulin. The rapid-acting analogues Aspart/Novolog, Gluisine/Apidra, and Lispro/Humalog have an onset of action ranging from 5 to 15 minutes; peak action occurs one hour after injection, and their duration of action is up to 4 hours. The rapid-acting analogues are typically administered before meal or at the end of the meal for the hospitalized patient as nutritional insulin to prevent hypoglycemia. Regular insulin has an onset of action of 30 to 45 minutes, peaks at 2 to 4 hours, and duration of up to 6 to 10 hours. Because of the delay of onset of action, regular insulin is challenging to match to nutritional intake in the hospital setting. Its longer duration of action may provide adequate coverage in some patients. Regular insulin is commonly used in insulin drips, insulin pumps, and sliding scale use. See **Table 2** for the types of insulin.

COMMON INSULIN REGIMENS IN THE HOSPITAL

On completion of assessment and identification of hyperglycemia, the initiation of the insulin regimen should be tailored to the specific patient and medical history. Individualized care will be more effective to manage the blood glucose level to prevent glucose excursions. In patients with T2DM, the Endocrine Society recommends the discontinuation of most oral and noninsulin injectable diabetes medications while hospitalized and switching the patient to a scheduled basal-bolus insulin regimen

Table 2	
Factors contributing to the development of hyperglycemia and hypoglycemia in hospitalized patients	
Hyperglycemia	**Hypoglycemia**
• Increased secretion of counterregulatory hormones secondary to physiologic stress	• Prolonged NPO status
• Infection	• Poor appetite
• Acute illness	• Malnutrition
• Surgery	• Severe liver disease
• Nutrition	• Renal insufficiency
• Parental Nutrition	
• Enteral nutrition	
• IV dextrose	
• Use of medications that cause hyperglycemia	
• Omitted insulin doses	
• Late insulin doses	
• Use of sliding scale insulin regimens only	
• Decreased exercise	
• Inadequate knowledge of the management of hyperglycemia and diabetes by health care providers	

while hospitalized. The prolonged use of sliding scale insulin therapy should be avoided because it increases the risk for hypoglycemia and hyperglycemia.[14] Many different regimens exist that are successful. The Endocrine Society recommends calculating the total daily insulin dose based on the following: if a patient is older than 69 years and/or the glomerular filtration rate (GFR) is less than 60 mL/min, multiply the kilograms of body weight by 0.2 to 0.3; if the patient is younger than 69 years and has a GFR of 60 or higher and the blood glucose level is 140 to 200 mg/dL, multiply the kilograms of body weight by 0.4; and if the patient is younger than 69 years and has a GFR of 60 or higher and the blood glucose level is 201 to 400 mg/dL, multiply the kilograms of body weight by 0.5.[8] The total daily dose is then distributed as approximately 50% basal and 50% bolus. The basal insulin is given as once daily glargine or twice daily NPH or detemir insulin. The total bolus dose is divided into 3 doses for the meals, and rapid-acting insulin is used. If the patient misses a meal, the meal dose is not given. Correction doses are calculated based on how sensitive the patient is to insulin. Patients who use more than 80 units per day or are receiving corticosteroids are insulin-resistant and those who are not eating, elderly, or have impaired renal function are insulin-sensitive. All others have usual sensitivity. If the patient develops hypoglycemia using one column, then switch the patient to a more sensitive column. If the patient develops hypoglycemia on the sensitive column, then adjust the doses for the column. If the patient is eating, then the bolus insulin dose using a rapid-acting insulin will cover the meal, and the correction is added to the meal dose if the blood glucose level is more than 140 mg/dL. If the patient is not eating, then the blood glucose is checked every 4 to 6 hours and regular insulin is given to correct hyperglycemia (**Table 3**).

Hospitalized patients with T1DM should always continue basal insulin therapy even if not eating to prevent DKA.[8] Most patients with T1DM use intensive insulin management at home before admission using multiple daily injections or an insulin pump. Patients with T1DM are usually more sensitive to insulin and require less insulin than those with T2DM. Recommendations for hospitalized patients with T1DM include the administration of long-acting basal insulin along with rapid-acting analogue therapy. Some hospitals have policies in place to allow the patient using an insulin pump to remain on the insulin pump during the hospital stay. The Endocrine Society recommends using a basal-bolus regimen similar to that used in T2DM, keeping in mind that the total daily dose may be less than that of patients with T2DM and that basal insulin is always required.

For patients with hyperglycemia secondary to glucocorticoid use, the Endocrine Society recommends bedside glucose monitoring in those who do not have a history of diabetes.[8] They recommend discontinuing bedside glucose monitoring if all blood glucose results are less than 140 mg/dL for 24 to 48 hours after discontinuation of the glucocorticoids. They recommend the initiation of a basal-bolus insulin regimen in patients with persistent hyperglycemia.

IMPLICATIONS FOR NURSING CARE OF HOSPITALIZED PATIENTS WITH HYPERGLYCEMIA AND DIABETES

The Joint Commission on Accreditation of Health care Organizations mandate for early discharge planning impresses the importance of the nurse providing the appropriate nursing interventions to prevent extreme glucose excursions.[15] Hospitals need to identify the role of the nurse in the management of blood glucose level with the hospitalized patient. Caring for patients with diabetes and hyperglycemia is challenging for the nurse. The nurse needs to monitor blood glucose level closely

Table 3
Types of insulin

	Types of Insulin	Onset	Peak	Duration	Appearance	Typical Use
Rapid-acting analogue (Bolus)	Aspart (Novolog) Lispro (Humalog) Glulisine (Apidra)	<15 min	0.5–1.5 h	3–4 h	clear	Premeals/correction of hyperglycemia
Short	Regular	0.5–1 h	2–3 h	3–6 h	clear	Correction of hyperglycemia
Intermediate	NPH	2–4 h	7–8 h	>10 h	Milky	Usually 2 doses per day with morning and evening meal.
Long (Basal)	Detemir (Levemir)	1–2 h	Flat, minimal or no peak	Up to 24 h	clear	Usually 1 dose at bedtime but may be divided 2 doses morning and bedtime.
	Glargine (Lantus)	1.5 h	Flat, minimal or no peak	Up to 24 h	clear	Usually 1 dose per day, either morning or bedtime.
Premixed insulins:	70/30 (70% NPH + 30% regular)	0.5–1 h	2–10 h	10–18 h	Milky	Usually dosed 2 times daily
	50/50 (50% NPH + 50% Regular)	0.5–1 h	2–10 h	10–18 h	Milky	
	Humalog Mix 75/25 (75% lispro protamine + 25% lispro)	10–15 min	1–3 h	10–16 h	Clear	
	Humalog Mix 50/50 (50% lispro proamine + 50% lispro)	10–15 min	1–3 h	10–16 h	Clear	
	Novolog Mix 70/30 (70% aspart protamine, 30% aspart)	10–20 min	1–4 h	10–16 h	Clear	

and respond quickly to hypoglycemia and hyperglycemia. The patient's nutrition intake needs to be monitored and insulin doses need to be given at the prescribed times. Basal insulin should not be withheld for NPO status unless orders are received to hold the basal insulin for NPO status. Documentation by the nurse includes the date, time, and result of the blood glucose tests, insulin doses given, insulin doses refused or held, and nutrition intake. The nurse needs to notify the insulin prescriber if the patient is going to start glucocorticoids, if the glucocorticoid dose is changed or discontinued; if the diet orders have been changed; if the patient changes rooms (insulin orders are often discontinued if the patient is transferred to a new room), and if the patient is going home or transferring to another facility soon. If the patient has diabetes self-care knowledge deficits, the nurse will need to either teach the patient or work with a diabetes educator to make sure that either the patient and/or another caregiver is able to perform all diabetes self-care skills after discharge. Hospitals should have policies and procedures guiding the care of the hospitalized patient with hyperglycemia and diabetes. See the Sample Insulin Use Guideline.

SUMMARY

Insulin is the most commonly used medication to manage hyperglycemia and diabetes in hospitalized patients. The appropriate use of insulin will control and prevent glucose excursions. Understanding the relationship of the action, peak, and duration of the different types of insulin will assist in the development of an individualized care plan to assist the patient not only in inpatient blood glucose level management but also in self-management care after discharge. Evidence-based standards of care related to the prevention and treatment of extreme manifestations of glycemic control includes the individualized and appropriate use of insulin related to action, peak, and duration. Hyperglycemia is a potent and independent risk factor for adverse outcomes for patients in the acute care. In an effort to improve patient safety, establishing a protocol for staff nurses and other health care professionals will decrease adverse outcomes, length of stay, and cost of care.

REFERENCES

1. National Institute of Diabetes and Digestive and Kidney Diseases. National diabetes statistics, 2011. Available at: http://www.diabetes.niddk.nih.gov/dm/pubs/statistics/#fast. Accessed August 20, 2012.
2. Centers for Disease Control and Prevention. 2011 National Diabetes Fact Sheet. Available at: http://www.dcd.gov/diabetes/pubs/estimates11htm. Accessed August 20, 2012.
3. McDonnell M, Umpierrez G. Insulin therapy for the management of hyperglycemia in hospitalized patients. Endocrinol Metab Clin North Am 2012;41: 175–201.
4. Umpierrez G, Isaac S, Bazargan H, et al. Hyperglycemia: an independent marker of in-hospital mortality in patients with undiagnosed diabetes. J Clin Endocrinol Metab 2006;87:978–82.
5. Olson L, Muchmore J, Lawrence C. The benefits of inpatient diabetes care: Improving quality of care and the bottom line. Endocr Pract 2006;12:35–42.
6. Mensing C, Boucher J, Cypress M, et al. National standards for diabetes self-management education. Diabetes Care 2006;29(Suppl 1):S78–85.

7. American Diabetes Association. Standards of medical care in diabetes-2012. Diabetes Care 2012;35:S11–63.
8. Umpierrez G, Hellman R, Kosiborod M, et al. Management of hyperglycemia in hospitalized patients in non-critical care setting: an endocrine society clinical practice guideline. J Clin Endocrinol Metab 2012;97:16–38.
9. Kitabchi A, Freire A, Umpierrez G. Evidence for strict inpatient blood glucose control: time to revise glycemic goals in hospitalized patients. Metabolism 2008;57:116–20.
10. American Diabetes Association. Position statement: standards of medical care in diabetes-2008. Available at: http://www.diabetes.org. Accessed August 20, 2012.
11. Bode B, Braithwaite S, Steed R, et al. Intravenous insulin infusion therapy: Indications, methods, and transition to subcutaneous insulin therapy. Endocr Pract 2004;10:71–80.
12. Van Den Berghe G, Wouters M, Wekers F, et al. Intensive insulin therapy in critically ill patients. N Engl J Med Nov 8 2001;345(19):1359–67.
13. Clement S, Braithwaite S, Magee M, et al. Management of diabetes and hyperglycemia in hospitals. Diabetes Care 2004;27:553–91.
14. Nau K, Lorenzetti R, Cucuzzella M, et al. Glycemic control in hospitalized patients not in intensive care: beyond sliding-scale insulin. Am Fam Physician 2010;81: 1130–5.
15. Joint Commission on Accreditation of Healthcare Organizations. National patient safety goals. Available at: http://www.jointcommission.org. Accessed August 20, 2012.

APPENDIX: SAMPLE INSULIN USE GUIDELINE
Purpose

To ensure safe administration of insulin and to explain the correct procedure for mixing of insulin types to eliminate multiple injections.

Policy

1. A physician's order is required for amount and types of insulin.
2. Sliding scale insulin orders are acceptable.
3. When documenting insulin administration, simultaneously record blood sugar values on the diabetes flow sheet and PCI (if appropriate).
4. Insulin shall never be diluted without consulting Pharmacy.
5. Mixed insulin should be given immediately.
6. Insulin is always to be given subcutaneously (SQ) unless ordered otherwise by physician.

Types of Insulin

Pharmacy will provide following types of insulin in FlexPen form if available from the manufacturer. Vials will be supplied to areas such as operating room and erectile dysfunction where vial use is more appropriate.

Insulin regular (Novolin R)
Insulin NPH (Novolin N)
Insulin NPH + Insulin regular mixture including Novolin 70/30 and Novolog 70/30
Insulin glargine (Lantus)

Insulin detemir (Levemir)
Insulin aspart (Novolog)
Insulin glulisine (Apidra)
Insulin aspart protamine + insulin aspart (Novolog Mix 70/30)

All Flexpens and Vials will have a 28-day Expiration Date Attached at the Time of Dispensing with the Exception of Novolog Mix 70/30, Which has a 14-day Expiration Date

General information

All insulin vials and prefilled insulin pens will be labeled with the patient's name and date opened and will remain in the patient's medication drawer.

- Under no circumstances are vials or prefilled pens of insulin to be "shared" among patients.

Subcutaneous administration sites will be documented in the medical record and on the diabetes flow sheet:

- Location of injection
- Time given
- Number of units
- Insulin type

Patients receiving intravenous total parenteral nutrition (TPN) therapy requiring insulin admixed into TPN fluid will receive regular insulin.

Mixtures of regular with NPH should be used within 5 minutes of mixing.

- The regular component takes on the characteristics of NPH after that time, and more of an NPH effect is obtained.
- Draw regular insulin into the syringe first and then draw up the NPH to prevent contamination of the regular insulin.

Glargine insulin and insulin detemir should not be mixed or diluted with any other form of insulin.

Timing of ordered dose:

- Aspart/lispro/glulisine insulin should be given within 15 minutes before a meal.
- Regular insulin is usually given 30 to 60 minutes before a meal.
- NPH insulin is usually dosed 1 to 2 times daily.
- Glargine (Lantus) insulin should be given at bedtime.
- Detemir (Levemir) is usually dosed once (with evening meal or at bedtime) or twice daily (with breakfast and then with evening meal or bedtime [12 hours apart]).

Insulin should not be frozen or exposed to high temperatures and direct light.

When a patient is switched from one purity to another, a dosage adjustment might be necessary, which cannot be predicted, and the dosage adjustment may be either up or down. The patient must be carefully monitored.

Hold Insulin

If patient's status is NPO, without any source of feeding (eg, tube feed or TPN), hold any insulin order; do not give any insulin without consulting physician.

Procedure

1. Validate order.
2. Identify patient using 2 identifiers.
3. Wash hands.
4. Confirm patient's blood sugar value (if appropriate).
5. If using vials, gather equipment:
   a. Prescribed insulin(s),
   b. Sterile alcohol wipes,
   c. Insulin syringe.
6. Draw up prescribed dosage of insulin in 100u/ml insulin syringe; verifying amount, type and expiration date of vial with another licensed nurse.
7. If mixing insulin types, draw up regular insulin first.
8. If using a FlexPen, the device should be primed per manufacturer's instructions before each injection to ensure accurate dosing.
9. Administer SQ unless physician orders alternative form.
10. Press site with alcohol wipe (do not rub). Rotate injection sites in and around previous injection sites to decrease variability in insulin absorption from dose to dose. The abdomen has the highest absorption rate, followed by the upper arm, thigh, and buttocks.

Equipments

Insulin vial
Insulin syringes
Prefilled insulin pens (FlexPen)
Alcohol swabs

Documentation

Document any patient family teaching in the patient care plan of the medical record and diabetes flow sheet.

Document the insulin administration in the medical record, the diabetes flow sheet, including the amount, type, and site of insulin administration along with current blood glucose level.

Patient/family teaching

Manufacturer's instructions for prefilled insulin pens and insulin self-administration process.

Sample Nutrition Guideline

Purpose

To establish guidelines for timing of blood glucose level monitoring and administering diabetes medications and/or insulin for hospitalized patients being served meals/snacks.

Procedure

A. Nursing personnel
   1. On a patient's admission, it is the responsibility of the nurse or patient care assistant to orient patient and family to the unit, including procedures for selecting menu, meal/snack delivery times, the timing of blood glucose checks, and timing of medications and/or insulin administration for their blood glucose analysis.
   2. It is the shared responsibility of the nursing personnel and the Food and Nutrition Service (FNS) staff to provide the appropriate menu to the patient.

3. It is the responsibility of the nursing personnel to coordinate with the patient when the patient selects his/her menu and check the patient's blood glucose level within 1 hour before meal and within 30 minutes before bedtime snack.
   - A key point to keep in mind is to discuss with the patients what time they last had food consumption. If patients ate within the previous 1 to 2 hours but is ready for their next meal, it is recommended that nurses document this to explain possible elevated blood glucose levels. This is also an opportunity to educate patients about the effects of food on blood glucose level and the importance of eating meals/snacks on a regular schedule as much as possible.
   - For those patients who are unable to select their own meals/snacks because of language barrier or cognition, it is the shared responsibility of the nursing personnel and FNS staff to provide an interpreter or arrange for selection of meals or snacks for these patients.
4. It is the responsibility of the nurse to medicate the patient for the blood glucose analysis within the appropriate time of the patient's meal or snack and document in the medical administration record (MAR)/diabetes flow sheet. If the time of the actual administration of the medication/insulin is not as printed on the MAR, document the reason as "meal time adjustment" or another reason as appropriate.
   - Keep in mind that the times printed on the MAR for insulin and other glucose lowering medications are only there as reminders that the medication/insulin is due to be given and may not necessarily reflect the true time to be administered. Make sure to document the appropriate reason for any deviations from the printed times.
   - This is another opportunity to educate patients about the effects of their medications and the importance of correct timing of medications and food.
5. It is the responsibility of the nursing staff to verify that the patient has received their meal or snack as appropriate. The bedtime snacks will be delivered to the unit by FNS staff. Nursing staff are responsible for delivering the snack to each patient identified with hyperglycemia/diabetes after blood glucose levels have been checked. Nursing staff need to verify that the patient has received the snack and encourage them to eat it, especially if they were medicated for their blood glucose analysis.
6. It is the responsibility of the nurse to notify the diabetes educator or the dietitian if a consult is needed for the patient. Document any interventions.

B. FNS personnel
   1. It is a shared responsibility of the FNS staff to ensure that the patient is aware of how to select choices on menu and that the patient has an appropriate menu. For those patients who are unable to select their menu because of language barrier or cognition, it is also the responsibility of the FNS staff to provide an interpreter or arrange for preselected meals for these patients.
   2. It is the responsibility of the FNS department to remind patients ordering from American Diabetes Association or No Concentrated Sweets menu to inform their nurse or patient care assistant that they have received their meal so that nursing staff can check blood glucose level and administer medication, as ordered by physician.
   3. It is also the responsibility of the FNS personnel to place a reminder card on the patients' trays to remind patients to notify their nurse or PCA to check blood glucose level and administer medication.

4. It is the responsibility of the FNS staff to ensure that patients receive their meals and snacks in a timely manner. If a delay is anticipated, FNS staff is to notify the nursing staff.

Equipment
Blood glucose meter.

Patient/family teaching/discharge planning
Meal planning and schedule, snack schedule, timing of prescribed diabetes medications, blood glucose monitoring schedule.

Documentation
Diabetes flow sheet, eMAR, meditech patient record, interdisciplinary plan of care, patient menu.

Unit	Tray Assembly Time	Tray Delivery Range
Breakfast		
Tower	7:15–7:25	7:30–7:45
600	7:25–7:35	7:40–7:55
700	7:35–7:45	7:50–8:05
1000	7:45–7:50	8:00–8:10
ICU	7:50–8:00	8:05–8:20
200	8:00–8:10	8:15–8:30
300	8:10–8:20	8:25–8:40
400	8:20–8:30	8:35–8:50
Lunch		
ICU	11:15–11:25	11:30–11:45
Tower	11:25–11:35	11:40–11:55
600	11:35–11:45	11:50–12:05
700	11:45–11:50	12:00–12:10
1000	11:50–12:00	12:05–12:20
200	12:00–12:10	12:15–12:30
300	12:10–12:20	12:25–12:40
400	12:20–12:30	12:35–12:50
Dinner		
ICU	4:15–4:25	4:30–4:45
Tower	4:25–4:35	4:40–4:55
600	4:35–4:45	4:50–5:05
700	4:45–4:50	5:00–5:10
1000	4:50–4:00	5:05–5:20
200	5:00–5:10	5:15–5:30
300	5:10–5:20	5:25–5:40
400	5:20–5:30	5:35–5:50

(Continued on next page)

Late tray cut off times:

Hot breakfast until 9 AM
Hot lunch until 1:30 PM
Hot dinner until 6 PM

Diet guidelines controlled diets that inpatient can order
Carbohydrate controlled Who is it for: Patients with hyperglycemia or a diagnosis of diabetes.

What is it: Restricted in simple sugars and carbohydrate foods.

1 Carbohydrate choice = 15 g carbohydrate.

Why do they need it: To control blood sugar levels by providing a consistent amount of carbohydrates at each meal and snack and limiting simple sugars.

Foods not recommended

- Sugar
- Regular maple syrup
- Regular jelly
- Regular gelatin
- Regular soda

Carbohydrate choices per meal depend on the calorie level:

Calorie Level	1200	1400	1600	1800	2000	2200	2400
Breakfast	2	2	3	4	4	4	5
10 AM Snack	1	1	1	1	1	1	2
Lunch	2	3	3	4	4	5	5
Dinner	3	3	4	4	5	5	5
HS Snack	1	1–2	1–2	1–2	1–2	1–2	1–2
Total Daily CHO	9	11	13	15	16	17	19

Snacks		
	10 AM	HS
Monday	Graham crackers-2 packets	1/2 cup cottage cheese and 1/2 cup fruit
Tuesday	Fruit cup-1	1 peanut butter and 2 pkg crackers
Wednesday	Sugar free pudding (vanilla)-1	2 oz cheese and 2 pkg crackers
Thursday	Applesauce-1	Sugar free pudding (chocolate)-1
Friday	Pretzels-1 bag	6 oz low fat yogurt
Saturday	Fruit cup-1	1/2 sandwich
Sunday	Whole wheat crackers-2 packets	6 oz low fat yogurt

Inpatient Diabetes Care

Word Search with a Hidden Message

```
B G L T O P R E V M E N T P N O D O A N E R O A O U T C O M O E S I
B I Y I M A D S A L N N A G I N G N L I A N M P S I T P T A O T T I E N
T U I B B E L L O CIR O N D V U G L U S C E T C O A S E I M E Y E E J
O S H N M T N Y O E N K M S E V W X I I T N I F E U L G M R C O H Y S
E G B C C T F S S J G I F K O I A W H N N V Z I A O A E F O O O T M S P N
J P A T U L H G X D P P I G O M Z V T Y G Y C D W D N J U W Y D N E U P
A U H Y R F K K Y I C C D H C I E N Y J S L U V H I S A M J A I T Y M W I I
L E V E M I R T C I F T F N M I J C K C F T F E A C D O T Y I F E K T G A V
J T W S B Q L O W N A O G V J S X T G J W L E K I T O V V C N T E C V E I
P N T D V N X G T G W P L N R R P K O E Q G D H O W E R C A M B B P D
A O N J W W D O S O S G R V N S B Y A G A T N E M S S E S S A G N I S R U N
```

BEDTIME SNACKS	COMMUNICATION	LEVEMIR
DIABETES EDUCATION	HUMALOG	LANTUS
TIMING OF MEALS	NOVOLOG	INSULIN
MONITORING	NOTIFY PHYSICIAN	
NURSING ASSESSMENT	PREVENT HYPOGLYCEMIA	
PREVENT DKA	SATISFIED PATIENTS	

_T_ _o_ _p_ _r_ _e_ _v_ _e_ _n_ _t_   _p_ _o_ _o_ _r_   _o_ _u_ _t_ _c_ _o_ _m_ _e_ _s_
_b_ _y_   _m_ _a_ _n_ _a_ _g_ _i_ _n_ _g_   _i_ _n_ _p_ _a_ _t_ _i_ _e_ _n_ _t_
_b_ _l_ _o_ _o_ _d_   _g_ _l_ _u_ _c_ _o_ _s_ _e_

Becky Childers RN, BSN, CDE

Created by Puzzlemaker at DiscoveryEducation.com

Procedure Skills Checklist

Procedure: Demonstration and Return Demonstration Training for the Novo Nordisk Insulin FlexPen®.

Employee Name: _____

Job Title: _____ Department/Unit: _____

PROCEDURE: PERFORM THE FOLLOWING:	MET	NOT MET
INSULIN INJECTION USING THE NOVO NORDISK INSULIN FlexPen®:		
1. Wash hands.		
2. Remove cap and wipe rubber stopper with alcohol pad.		
3. For Novolog Mix 70/30, roll FlexPen® between palms 10 times prior to use. No rolling necessary for clear insulin.		
4. If less than 12 units left in the Novolog Mix 70/30 FlexPen®, please do not use.		
5. Remove the protective cap from the Novofine autocover disposable safety needle and, with the needle pointing away from you, screw it tightly on to the pen.		

(continued on next page)

PERFORM THE AIRSHOT:		
1. Turn the dial to 2 units. (Prime according to manufacturer's instructions)		
2. Point needle upward and tap reservoir gently with finger a few times; remove the needle cap.		
3. With needle still upward, press the push button as far as it will go until you visualize a drop of insulin at the needle tip (this is an airshot).		
4. If you do not see a drop, perform another airshot, if no drop appears after 6 airshots, do not use the insulin pen and return it to the Pharmacy.		
SETTING THE DOSE:		
1. Verify dose selector set at zero.		
2. Dial the number of units of insulin ordered.		
3. Verify the number of units with a second licensed staff.		
GIVING THE INJECTION:		
1. Choose the injection site. Wipe with alcohol pad.		
2. Pinch up the skin.		
3. Turn the Dose Indicator Window of the pen so that it faces you.		
4. Push the NovoFine autocover disposable safety needle shield against the skin and allow the needle to enter the skin. Visually verify that the sliding needle shield is retracted, and the needle hub is against the skin.		
5. Press the button all the way in and keep the needle in for at least 6 seconds to make sure all the insulin injects.		
6. Keep the push button fully depressed until the needle is withdrawn from the skin.		
7. Withdraw the needle and ensure the safety lock has engaged. (Red indicator should be visible.)		
8. Do not recap the needle and dispose of the needle into the sharps box.		
9. Replace the cap on the Novo Nordisk FlexPen® for storage.		
PATIENT DISCHARGE INSTRUCTIONS:		
1. Instruct the patient on use of FlexPen® as ordered by prescribing physician prior to discharge.		
2. Physician to provide a written prescription to include FlexPen® and needle tips.		

NOTE: DEMONSTRATE COMPETENCY UNDER DIRECT OBSERVATION OF PRECEPTOR WITH 100% ACCURACY.

o Passed	o Repeat

Signature: _____

Oriented/Validated by: _____

Completion Date: _____

2010, Becky Childers RN, BSN, CDE referenced from Novo Nordisk, Inc. Training for the Novo Nordisk Insulin FlexPen.

Management of Hypertension in Patients with Diabetes

Celia M. Levesque, RN, MSN, NP-C, CNS-BC, BC-ADM, CDE

KEYWORDS

- Diabetes • Hypertension • Cardiovascular disease • Antihypertension medication

KEY POINTS

- Hypertension is a major contributing factor to the development of cardiovascular disease, especially in patients with diabetes.
- The management of hypertension in patients with diabetes is equally important as glucose control in the prevention of long-term diabetes complications.
- It is important to treat patients with hypertension who have diabetes according to evidence-based medicine and national guidelines.

INTRODUCTION

Mortality from cardiovascular disease is 2 to 4 times higher in patients with type 2 diabetes compared with patients with similar demographic characteristics but without diabetes.[1] Hypertension is a major contributing factor to the development of cardiovascular disease. The management of hypertension in patients with diabetes is as important as glucose control to the prevention and management of long-term diabetes complications. This article discusses the incidence of hypertension in diabetes, the impact of hypertension on the development of long-term complications, diagnosis of hypertension in patients with diabetes, blood pressure goals, the treatment of hypertension in patients with diabetes, and antihypertension medications.

INCIDENCE OF HYPERTENSION IN DIABETES

According to the American Diabetes Association, 2 out of 3 adults with diabetes have high blood pressure.[1] The incidence and presentation of hypertension is different in patients with type I diabetes compared with type 2 diabetes.[2] In patients with type I diabetes, hypertension is usually the result of underlying nephropathy, whereas patients with type 2 diabetes usually have hypertension that coexists with other

Department of Endocrine Neoplasia and Hormonal Disorders, The University of Texas MD Anderson Cancer Center, PO Box 301402, Unit 1461, Houston, TX 77230-1402, USA
E-mail address: clevesqu@mdanderson.org

Crit Care Nurs Clin N Am 25 (2013) 71–91
http://dx.doi.org/10.1016/j.ccell.2012.11.008
0899-5885/13/$ – see front matter © 2013 Elsevier Inc. All rights reserved.
ccnursing.theclinics.com

cardiometabolic risk factors. Patients with type I diabetes generally develop hypertension after several years of having the disease. The incidence of hypertension in patients with type I diabetes is 5% after having the disease for 10 years; after 20 years, the incidence increases to 33%; and after 40 years, the incidence increases to 70%.[3] The incidence of hypertension in patients with type 2 diabetes is 1.5 to 3 times higher than in people without diabetes in age-matched groups.[2]

THE IMPACT OF HYPERTENSION ON THE DEVELOPMENT OF LONG-TERM DIABETES COMPLICATIONS

Hypertension is a major contributor for cardiovascular events including myocardial infarction and stroke.[3] It is also a risk factor for microvascular complications including retinopathy and nephropathy. Cardiovascular disease is the most common cause of death in patients with diabetes. It is thought to account for 86% of all deaths of patients with diabetes. See **Box 1** for the major cardiovascular risk factors in patients with diabetes. An increase in diastolic or systolic blood pressure of 5 mm Hg is associated with a concomitant increase in cardiovascular disease of 20% to 30%. If the diastolic blood pressure is greater than 70 mm Hg, retinopathy progresses at a faster rate.

Hypertension is approximately 2 times higher in patients with diabetes compared with patients without diabetes.[4] In patients with diabetes, 75% of all cardiovascular disease is attributable to hypertension. The current recommendation is to reduce blood pressure to less than 130/85 mm Hg.

The risk factors for the development of hypertension in patients with diabetes include the development of diabetic nephropathy, hyperinsulinemia, extracellular fluid volume expansion, and increased arterial stiffness. Microalbuminuria and macroalbuminuria is a risk factor for the development of hypertension in patients with type I diabetes. A study of 981 patients with type I diabetes for 5 or more years showed that hypertension was present in 19% of patients with normoalbuminuria, 30% of patients with microalbuminuria, and 65% of patients with macroalbuminuria.[5] The incidence of

---

Box 1
Major cardiovascular risk factors in patients with diabetes

- Hypertension
- Age (older than 55 years for men, 65 years for women)
- Diabetes mellitus
- Increased low-density lipoprotein (LDL)
- Increased total cholesterol,
- Low high-density lipoprotein (HDL) cholesterol
- Estimated glomerular filtration rate (eGFR) less than 60 mL/min
- Family history of premature cardiovascular disease (men less than 55 years of age or women less than 65 years of age)
- Microalbuminuria
- Obesity (body mass index [BMI] >30 kg/m^2)
- Physical inactivity
- Tobacco usage, particularly cigarettes

hypertension in patients with progressive diabetic nephropathy is approximately 75% to 85%.[6]

Hyperinsulinemia develops secondary to insulin resistance in patients with type 2 diabetes.[6] Hyperinsulinemia may increase systemic blood pressure. The blood pressure may also increase after initiating exogenous insulin therapy. It is not understood whether the exogenous insulin increases the blood pressure directly or the concomitant weight gain that usually accompanies insulin initiation causes the increased blood pressure. Hypertension is linked with obesity in patients with and without diabetes. Insulin may increase sympathetic activity and promote renal sodium retention. The excess glucose is reabsorbed in the proximal tubule through the sodium-glucose cotransporter and causes an increase in sodium reabsorption. Sodium retention causes volume expansion, which increases blood pressure. Increased arterial stiffness caused by protein glycation causes an increase in systolic blood pressure and is linked with an increased mortality risk.[7]

DIAGNOSING HYPERTENSION IN PATIENTS WITH DIABETES

The blood pressure should be measured at every diabetes visit.[1] The blood pressure at the office should be measured by a trained professional when patients are seated with their feet on the floor and their arms supported at the heart level. The patient should rest for 5 minutes before taking the blood pressure. The cuff size should be appropriate for the upper arm circumference. See **Box 2** for accurate measurement of blood pressure. If the systolic blood pressure is equal to or greater than 130 mm Hg or the diastolic blood pressure equal to or greater than 80 mm Hg the blood pressure should be taken on a separate day to make a diagnosis of hypertension. See **Table 1** for the diagnosis of hypertension.

Box 2
Accurate blood pressure measurement

- The auscultatory method of blood pressure measurement should be used.

- Persons should be seated quietly for at least 5 minutes in a chair (rather than on an examination table), with feet on the floor, and the arm supported at heart level.

- Caffeine, exercise, and smoking should be avoided for at least 30 minutes before measurement.

- Measurement of blood pressure in the standing position is indicated periodically, especially in those at risk for postural hypotension, before a necessary drug dose or adding a drug, and in those who report symptoms consistent with reduced blood pressure on standing.

- An appropriately sized cuff (cuff bladder encircling at least 80% of the arm) should be used to ensure accuracy.

- At least 2 measurements should be made and the average recorded.

- For manual determinations, a palpated radial pulse obliteration pressure should be used to estimate systolic blood pressure and the cuff should then be inflated to 20 to 30 mm Hg more than this level. The cuff deflation rate should be 2 mm Hg per second.

- Systolic blood pressure is the point at which the first of 2 or more Korotkoff sounds is heard (onset of phase 1), and the disappearance of Korotkoff sound (onset of phase 5) is used to define diastolic blood pressure.

- Clinicians should provide to patients, verbally and in writing, the patients' specific blood pressure numbers and the blood pressure goal of their treatment.

| Table 1 |
| Diagnosis of hypertension |

Blood Pressure Classification	Systolic Blood Pressure (mm Hg)	Diastolic Blood Pressure (mm Hg)
Normal	<120	And <80
Prehypertension	120–139	Or 80–89
Stage 1 hypertension	140–159	Or 90–99
Stage 2 hypertension	>160	Or >100

BLOOD PRESSURE GOAL

Because of the complications caused by high blood pressure in people with diabetes, the American Diabetes Association and the National Institutes of Health recommend a lower blood pressure target than for the general population.[1,2] They recommend a blood pressure goal of less than 130/80 mm Hg. The Action to Control Cardiovascular Disease and Diabetes (ACCORD) was a randomized, multicenter, 2-by-2 factorial trial involving 10,251 patients with type 2 diabetes.[8] The purpose of this study was to examine the effects of intensive glycemic control, fibrate treatment to increase HDL-cholesterol (HDL-C) and lower triglycerides, and intensive blood pressure control on cardiovascular outcomes. A total of 4733 participants with type 2 diabetes were randomly assigned to blood pressure management with a systolic blood pressure target of less than 120 mm Hg or standard therapy with a systolic blood pressure target of less than 140 mm Hg. After 1 year, the mean systolic blood pressure was 119.3 mm Hg in the intensive therapy group and 133.5 mm Hg in the standard therapy group. The annual death rate from any cause was 1.8% in the intensive group and 1.19% in the standard group. The annual rate of stroke was 0.32% in the intensive group and 0.53% in the standard group. Adverse events attributed to antihypertensive treatment occurred in 77 of the 2362 participants in the intensive therapy group and 30 of the 2371 participants in the standard group. The conclusion was that achieving a systolic blood pressure of less than 120 mm Hg in patients with type 2 diabetes did not reduce the rate of fatal and nonfatal major cardiovascular events compared with the standard group with a target of less than 140 mm Hg.

The Action in Diabetes and Vascular Disease: Preterax and Diamicron MR Controlled Evaluation (ADVANCE) trial was a randomized multicenter trial in 20 countries involving 11,140 patients with type 2 diabetes who were older than 55 years and developed type 2 diabetes after the age of 30 years.[9] The patients were required to have a history of a major cardiovascular disease event including stroke, myocardial infarction, hospital admission for transient ischemic attack, hospital admission for unstable angina, coronary revascularization, peripheral revascularization, amputation secondary to vascular disease, or at least 1 other risk factor for cardiovascular disease. The risk factors included a minimum of 1 of the following: a history of major microvascular disease including macroalbuminuria, proliferative diabetic retinopathy, retinal photocoagulation therapy, macular edema, or blindness in 1 eye thought to be caused by diabetes, current cigarette smoking, total cholesterol more than 6.0 mmol (232 mg/dL), HDL cholesterol less than 1.0 mmol (38 mg/dL), microalbuminuria, diagnosis of type 2 diabetes greater than 10 years before entry into the study, or age 65 years or older at the entry of the study. Treatment with an angiotensin-converting enzyme inhibitor (ACEI) and a thiazide-type diuretic reduced the rate of death but not the composite macrovascular outcome. The mean systolic blood pressure in the intensive group was 135 mm Hg.

The International Verapamil SR/Trandolapril Study (INVEST) trial was a prospective, randomized, open, blinded end point trial that involved 22,576 patients aged 50 years or older who had diabetes and coexisting coronary artery disease.[10] In addition to hypertension and coronary artery disease, most patients had 1 or more risk factors including diabetes, dyslipidemia, prior history of smoking, or a history of being overweight or obese. The results suggested that controlling blood pressure to the goal of less than 130 mm Hg was not associated with improved cardiovascular outcome compared with the usual care. The American Diabetes Association, based on the study results of the ACCORD, ADVANCE, and INVEST trials, therefore recommends that systolic blood pressure should be managed at less than 130 mm Hg for most patients.[1]

TREATMENT OF HYPERTENSION IN PATIENTS WITH DIABETES

Early and aggressive treatment of hypertension is vital to help reduce the risk of cardiovascular disease, renal disease, retinopathy, and other microvascular and macrovascular disease in patients with diabetes. After the diagnosis of hypertension is made, a decision has to be made for whether the patient should be given a chance to make therapeutic lifestyle changes to improve blood pressure without the use of antihypertensive medications, or whether antihypertensive medication is needed immediately. That decision is based on the blood pressure at diagnosis.[1,11] If the systolic blood pressure is 130 to 139 mm Hg or if the diastolic blood pressure is 80 to 89 mm Hg, the patient may be given a chance to improve blood pressure via therapeutic lifestyle changes alone. Therapeutic lifestyle changes include weight loss if the patient is overweight, the Dietary Approaches to Stop Hypertension (DASH) diet, sodium restriction of less than 1500 mg per day, increased potassium intake, moderation of alcohol intake, and increased physical activity, low-fat dairy products, and 8 to 10 servings per day. Alcohol consumption should be limited to no more than 2 drinks per day in men and no more than 1 drink per day in women. See **Table 2** for the effects of therapeutic lifestyle changes on blood pressure. See **Box 3** for the DASH eating plan.

If the systolic blood pressure is greater than 139 mm Hg or the diastolic blood pressures is greater than 89 mm Hg, antihypertensive medication should be initiated in addition to therapeutic lifestyle changes.[1] Before starting antihypertensive medications,

Table 2
Effect of therapeutic lifestyle changes on blood pressure

Modification	Recommendation	Approximate Systolic Blood Pressure Reduction Range (mm Hg)
Weight reduction	Maintain normal body weight (BMI 18.5–24.9)	5–20/10 kg weight lost
Adopt DASH eating plan	Diet rich in fruits, vegetables, low-fat dairy items, and reduced in other fats	8–14
Restrict sodium intake	<2.4 g of sodium per day	2–8
Physical activity	Regular aerobic exercise for at least 30 minutes on most days of the week	4–9
Moderate alcohol consumption	<2 drinks/d for men and <1 drink/d for women	2–4

Box 3
DASH eating plan

- Rich in fruits, vegetables, and low-fat dairy products
- Reduced content of dietary cholesterol as well as saturated and total fat
- Rich in potassium and calcium content
- Dietary sodium should be reduced to no more than 100 mmol per day (2.4 g of sodium)
- Alcohol intake should be limited to:
  - No more than 30 mL (1 oz) of ethanol
  - Equivalent of 2 drinks per day in most men
  - Equivalent of 1 drink per day in women and lighter weight persons
  - A drink is 355 ml (12 oz) of beer, 150 mL (5 oz) of wine, and 45 mL (1.5 oz) of 80-proof liquor

---

12-lead electrocardiogram (ECG), urinalysis, blood glucose, hematocrit, serum potassium, creatinine, glomerular filtration rate (GFR), calcium, lipid panel, urinary albumin, and other tests should be performed if a secondary cause of hypertension is suspected.[11] See **Box 4** for routine tests and procedures to be done before hypertension treatment. Antihypertensive medications for people with diabetes should include a regimen that includes an ACEI or an angiotensin receptor blocker (ARB).[1,11] Most patients require multiple drug therapy to control blood pressure. If an ACEI, ARB, or diuretic is used, the kidney function and serum potassium levels should be monitored. If the patient is pregnant, an ACEI, ARB, and many of the other antihypertensive medications cannot be used.

Choosing an initial monotherapy or combination therapy can be difficult. Many studies suggest that using an ACEI or ARB in patients with diabetes is a first-line treatment. The blood pressure arm of the ADVANCE trial showed that using a fixed combination of an ACEI (perindopril) and diuretic (indapamide) improved microvascular and macrovascular outcomes as well as cardiovascular disease and total mortality.[9] The

---

Box 4
Routine tests and procedures to be done before starting antihypertensive medications

- 12-lead ECG
- Urinalysis
- Blood glucose
- Hematocrit
- Serum potassium
- Creatinine (or the corresponding eGFR)
- Calcium
- Lipoprotein profile (after a 9-hour to 12-hour fast) that includes HDL-C, LDL-cholesterol, and triglycerides
- Urinary albumin excretion or albumin/creatinine ratio except for those with diabetes or kidney disease for whom annual measurements should be made
- Other tests as appropriate if the patient has an identifiable cause of hypertension

Avoiding Cardiovascular Events through Combination Therapy in Patients Living with Systolic Hypertension (ACCOMPLISH) trial showed that initial antihypertensive therapy with benazepril plus amlodipine was superior to the benazepril plus hydrochlorothiazide in reducing cardiovascular morbidity and mortality.[12] If additional medications are needed, amlodipine, hydrochlorothiazide, or chlorthalideone can be added.

The Seventh Report of the Joint National Committee on Prevention, Detection, Evaluation, and Treatment of High Blood Pressure (JNC7) recommends antihypertensive medications based on a combination of the stage of hypertension and whether or not the patient has compelling indications.[11] For patients with diabetes, they recommend using 1 or more of the following classes: diuretics, β-blockers (BB), ACEI, ARB, and calcium channel blocker (CCB). See **Table 3** for the JNC7 recommendations for initial medication for hypertension and **Table 4** for the JNC7 recommendations of antihypertension medication based on compelling indication.

If the blood pressure is not at target after using 3 antihypertensive medications from different drug classes, 1 of which is a diuretic, the clinician should consider evaluating for secondary forms of hypertension.[1] See **Box 5** for identifiable causes of hypertension and **Table 5** for the associated tests for identifiable causes of hypertension.

The American Diabetes Association recommends giving at least 1 of the antihypertensive medications at bedtime.[1] Most antihypertensive drugs are not safe during pregnancy. Drugs known to be effective and safe during pregnancy include methyldopa, labetalol, diltiazem, clonidine, and prazosin.

HYPERTENSION DRUG CLASSES

The most commonly used antihypertensive medication classes in patients with diabetes include ACEI, ARB, diuretics, CCB, and BB. When these classes do not control hypertension in patients with diabetes other classes may need to be added. These classes include α-adrenoreceptor antagonists, centrally acting sympatholytics, direct-acting vasodilators, nitrodilators, potassium channel openers, and renin inhibitors. See **Table 6** for antihypertensive medications and their associated classes.

ACEIs

Angiotensin II is a potent chemical that causes the muscles surrounding blood vessels to contract. The narrowed blood vessels cause the blood pressure to increase. Angiotensin II is formed from angiotensin I in the blood by the enzyme angiotensin-converting enzyme (ACE). ACEIs are medications that inhibit the activity of the enzyme ACE. Angiotensin-converting enzyme breaks down bradykinin. If bradykinin breakdown is blocked by the use of an ACEI, the increased bradykinin levels may cause the patient to have a dry cough. The ACEI produces vasodilatation by inhibiting the formation of angiotensin II. ACEIs are indicated for hypertension and heart failure. According to the JNC7, ACEIs have a compelling indication for use in patients with

Table 3
JNC7 recommendations for initial medication for hypertension

Without Compelling Indications		With Compelling Indications
Stage 1:	Stage 2:	Drug(s) for the compelling
Thiazide-type diuretics for most	2-drug combination for most	indications
	Usual: thiazide diuretic with	Other antihypertensive drugs
Consider ACEI ARB, BB, CCB, or combination	ACEI or ARB, or BB, or CCB	(diuretics, ACEI, ARB, BB, CCB) as needed

Table 4
JNC7 recommendations of antihypertension medication based on compelling indication

Compelling Indication	Diuretic	BB	ACEI	ARB	CCB	Aldo Ant
HF	X	X	X	X	X	X
After MI	—	X	X	—	—	X
High CAD risk	X	X	X	—	X	—
Diabetes	X	X	X	X	X	—
CKD	—	—	X	X	—	—
Recurrent CVA prevent	X	—	X	—	—	—

Abbreviations: Aldo Ant, aldosterone antagonist; CAD, coronary artery disease; CKD, chronic kidney disease; CVA, cerebral vascular accident; HF, heart failure; MI, myocardial infarction.

heart failure, status post myocardial infarction, coronary artery disease risk, diabetes, chronic kidney disease, and recurrent cerebral vascular accident prevention.[11] The most common side effects of ACEI include cough, increased serum potassium levels, hypotension, dizziness, headache, drowsiness, weakness, metallic or salty taste, and

Box 5
Identifiable causes of hypertension

- Chronic kidney disease
- Coarctation of the aorta
- Cushing syndrome and other glucocorticoid excess states including chronic steroid therapy
- Drug induced or drug related
- Nonadherence
- Inadequate doses
- Inappropriate combinations
- Nonsteroidal antiinflammatory drugs; cyclooxygenase-2 inhibitors
- Cocaine, amphetamines, other illicit drugs
- Sympathomimetics (decongestants, anorectics)
- Oral contraceptive hormones
- Adrenal steroid hormones
- Cyclosporine and tacrolimus
- Erythropoietin
- Licorice
- Some chewing tobacco
- Selected over-the-counter dietary supplements and medicines (eg, ephedra, ma huang, bitter orange)
- Obstructive uropathy
- Pheochromocytoma
- Primary aldosteronism and other mineralocorticoid excess states
- Renovascular hypertension
- Sleep apnea
- Thyroid or parathyroid disease

Table 5
Screening tests for identifiable hypertension

Diagnosis	Diagnostic Test
Chronic kidney disease	Estimated GFR
Coarctation of the aorta	CT angiography
Cushing syndrome and other glucocorticoid excess states, including chronic steroid therapy	History, dexamethasone suppression test
Drug induced/related	History; drug screening
Pheochromocytoma	24-h urinary metanephrine and normetanephrine
Primary aldosteronism and other mineralocorticoid excess states	24-h urinary aldosterone level or specific measurements of other mineralocorticoids
Renovascular hypertension	Doppler flow study; magnetic resonance angiography
Sleep apnea	Sleep study with O_2 saturation
Thyroid/parathyroid	TSH; serum PTH

Abbreviations: CT, computed tomography; PTH, parathyroid hormone; TSH, thyroid-stimulating hormone.

rash. Rare but serious side effects include angioedema, allergic reaction, and kidney failure. If an ACEI is used with patients with bilateral renal artery stenosis, renal failure may occur because increased circulating and intrarenal angiotensin II in this condition constricts the efferent arteriole more than the afferent arteriole within the kidney, which helps to maintain glomerular capillary pressure and filtration. This class of medication is contraindicated during pregnancy. Use caution with the elderly; the dose should be started low and titrated slow. Other precautions include use in patients with renal disease, concomitant use with potassium-sparing diuretics, potassium supplements, and/or potassium-containing salt substitutes.

ARBs

ARBs have a similar mechanism of action to ACEI and are used for the same indications (hypertension, heart failure, after myocardial infarction). They inhibit the formation of angiotensin II by blocking type 1 angiotensin II receptors on blood vessels and other tissues such as the heart. Because ARBs do not inhibit ACE, they do not cause an increase in bradykinin, which contributes to the vasodilatation produced by ACEI and some of the side effects of ACEI (cough and angioedema). This class dilates arteries and veins, reducing arterial pressure, preload, and afterload of the heart. They downregulate sympathetic adrenergic activity by blocking the effects of angiotensin II on sympathetic nerves and the release and reuptake of norepinephrine. They promote renal excretion of sodium and water by blocking the effects of angiotensin II in the kidney and by blocking angiotensin II stimulation of aldosterone secretion. They inhibit cardiac and vascular remodeling associated with chronic hypertension, heart failure, and myocardial infarction. As a class, ARBs have a low incidence of side effects and are generally well tolerated. They do not increase bradykinin levels like ACEI so they do not cause a cough or angioedema. Contraindications include pregnancy. Patients with bilateral renal artery stenosis may experience renal failure if ARBs are used.

Table 6
Antihypertensive medications and their associated drug classes

Name	Class	Dose Available (mg)
Accupril	ACEI	Quinapril HCl 5+, 10, 20, 40 tablets
Accuretic	ACEI and diuretic	Quinapril/HCTZ 10/12.5+, 20/12.5+, 20/25 tablets
Aceon	ACEI	Perindopril erbumine 2+, 4+, 8+ tablets
Adalat CC	CCB dihydropyridine	Nifedipine 30, 60, 90 ext-rel tablets
Afeditab CR	CCB dihydropyridine	Nifedipine 30, 60 ext-rel tablets
Aldactazide	Diuretic combination	Spironolactone/HCTZ 25/25, 50/50+ tablets
Aldactone	Diuretic K+ sparing	Spironolactone 25, 50+, 100+ tablets
Aldoril 15	Central α-agonist and diuretic	Methyldopa/HCTZ 250/15 tablets
Aldoril 25	Central α-agonist and diuretic	Methyldopa/HCTZ 250/25 tablets
Aldoril D30	Central α-agonist and diuretic	Methyldopa/HCTZ 500/30 tablets
Aldoril D50	Central α-agonist and diuretic	Methyldopa/HCTZ 500/50 tablets
Altace	ACEI	Ramipril 1.25, 2.5, 5, 10 gel caps
Amiloride	Diuretic K+ sparing	Amiloride HCl 5 tablets
Amiloride/HCTZ	Diuretic combination	Amiloride HCl/HCTZ 5/50+ tablets
Amturnide	Renin inhibitor, dihydropyridine CCB, and thiazide diuretic	Aliskiren hemifumarate/amlodipine besylate/HCTZ 150/5/12.5, 300/5/12.5, 300/5/25, 300/10/12.5, 300/10/25 tablets
Atacand	ARB	Candesartan cilexetil 4, 8, 16, 32 tablets
Atacand HCT	ARB and diuretic	Candesartan cilexetil/HCTZ 16/12.5, 32/12.5, 32/25 tablets
Avalide	ARB and diuretic	Irbesartan/HCTZ 150/12.5, 300/12.5 tablets
Avapro	ARB	Irbesartan 75, 150, 300 tablets
Azor	CCB and ARB	Amlodipine besylate/olmesartan medoxomil 5/20, 10/20, 5/40, 10/40 tablets
Benicar	ARB	Olmesartan medoxomil 5, 20, 40 tablets

(continued on next page)

Table 6
(continued)

Name	Class	Dose Available (mg)
Benicar HCT	ARB and diuretic	Olmesartan medoxomil/HCTZ 20/12.5, 40/12.5, 40/25 tablets
Bystolic	Cardioselective BB	Nebivolol (as HCl) 2.5, 5, 10 tablets
Caduet	CCB and HMG-CoA reductase inhibitor	Amlodipine besylate + atorvastatin 2.5/10, 2.5/20, 2.5/40, 5/10, 5/20, 5/40, 5/80, 10/10, 10/20, 10/40, 10/80 tablets
Calan	CCB diphenylalkylamine	Verapamil HCl 40, 80+, 120+ tablets
Calan SR	CCB diphenylalkylamine	Verapamil HCl 120, 180+, 240+, sus-rel caplets
Capoten	ACEI	Captopril 12.5+, 25+, 50+, 100+ tablets
Capozide	ACEI and diuretic	Captopril/HCTZ 25/15+, 25/25+, 50/15+, 50/25+ tablets
Cardene IV	CCB dihydropyridine	Nicardipine HCl 2.5/mL (after dilution to 0.1/mL) IV
Cardene IV premixed	CCB dihydropyridine	Nicardipine HCl 0.1/mL, 0.2/mL IV
Cardene SR	CCB dihydropyridine	Nicardipine HCl 30, 45, 60 sus-rel cap
Cardizem CD	CCB benzothiazepine	Diltiazem HCl 120, 180, 240, 300, 360 ext-rel cap
Cardizem LA	CCB benzothiazepine	Diltiazem HCl 120, 180, 240, 300, 360, 420 ext-rel cap
Cardura	α_1-blocker quinazoline	Doxazosin as mesylate 1+, 2+, 4+, 8+ tablets
Catapres	Central α-agonist	Clonidine HCl 0.1+, 0.2+, 0.3+ tablets
Catapres-TTS patch	Central α-agonist	Clonidine HCl 0.1/day, 0.2/day, 0.3/day, 1 patch/wk
Chlorothiazide	Diuretic thiazide	Chlorothiazide 250+, 500+ tablets
Chlorthalidone	Diuretic monosulfamyl	Chlorthalidone 25, 50 tablets
Cleviprex	CCB dihydropyridine	Clevidipine butyrate emulsion 0.5/mL IV
Coreg	Noncardioselective BB and α_1-blocker	Carvedilol 3.125, 6.25, 12.5, 25 tablets
Coreg CR	Noncardioselective BB and α_1-blocker	Carvedilol phosphate 10, 20, 40, 80 ext-rel cap

(continued on next page)

Table 6
(continued)

Name	Class	Dose Available (mg)
Corgard	Noncardioselective BB	Nadolol 20+, 40+, 80+, 120+, 160+ tablets
Corlopam	Dopamine D_1-like receptor agonist	Fenoldopam mesylate 10/mL IV
Corzide	Noncardioselective BB and diuretic	Nadolol/bendroflumethiazide 40/5+, 80/5+ tablets
Covera-HS	CCB diphenylalkylamine	Verapamil HCl 180, 240 controlled-onset ext-rel tablets
Cozaar	ARB	Losartan potassium 25, 50, 100 tablets
Demadex	Diuretic loop	Torsemide 5+, 10+, 20+, 100+ tablets
Demadex injection	Diuretic loop	Torsemide 10/mL IV
Demser	Tyrosine hydroxylase inhibitor	Metyrosine 250 caps
Dibenzyline	α-receptor blocker	Phenoxybenzamine HCl 10 caps
Dilacor XR	CCB benzothiazepine	Diltiazem HCl 120, 180, 240 ext-rel cap
Diovan	ARB	Valsartan 40+, 80, 160, 320 tablets
Diovan HCT	ARB and diuretic	Valsartan/HCTZ 80/12.5, 160/12.5, 160/25, 320/12.5, 320/25 tablets
Dutoprol	Cardioselective β1-blocker and diuretic	Metoprolol succinate ext-rel/HCTZ 25/12.5, 50/12.5, 100/12.5 tablets
Dyazide	Diuretic combination	Triamterene/HCTZ 37.5/25 caps
Dynacirc CR	CCB dihydropyridine	Isradipine 5, 10 controlled-release tablets
Edarbi	ARB	Azilsartan medoxomil 40, 80 tablets
Edarbyclor	ARB and diuretic	Azilsartan medoxomil/chlorthalidone 40/12.5, 40/25 tablets
Enalaprilat injection	ACEI	Enalaprilat 1.25/mL IV
Exforge	CCB and ARB	Amlodipine besylate/valsartan 5/160, 5/320, 10/160, 10/320 tablets

(continued on next page)

Table 6 (continued)		
Name	Class	Dose Available (mg)
Exforge HCT	CCB, ARB, and diuretic	Amlodipine besylate/valsartan/ HCTZ 5/160/12.5, 5/160/25, 10/160/ 12.5, 10/160/25, 10/320/25 tablets
Fosinopril	ACEI	Fosinopril sodium 10+, 20, 40 tablets
Fosinopril/HCTZ	ACEI and diuretic	Fosinopril sodium/HCTZ 10/12.5, 20/12.5 tablets
Hydralazine injection	Vasodilator	Hydralazine HCl 20/mL IM or IV
Hydralazine tablets	Vasodilator	Hydralazind HCl 10, 25, 50, 100 tablets
Hydrochlorothiazide	Diuretic thiazide	Hydrochlorothiazide 25+, 50+ tablets
Hytrin	α_1-blocker quinazoline	Terazosin HCl 1, 2, 5, 10 caps
Hyzaar	ARB and diuretic	Losartan potassium/HCTZ 50/12.5, 100/12.5, 100/25 tablets
Indapamide	Diuretic indoline	Indapamide 1.25, 2.5 tablets
Inderal	Noncardioselective BB	Propranolol HCl 10+, 20+, 40+, 60+ 80+ tablets
Inderal LA	Noncardioselective BB	Propranolol HCl 60, 80, 120, 160 sus-rel caps
Inderide	Noncardioselective BB and diuretic	Propranolol HCl/HCTZ 40/25+, 80/25+ tablets
Innopran XL	Noncardioselective BB	Propranolol HCl 80, 120 ext-rel caps
Inspra	Aldosterone receptor blocker mineralocorticoid selective	Eplerenone 25, 50 tablets
Isoptin SR	CCB diphenylalkylamine	Verapamil HCl 120, 180+, 240+, sus-rel tablets
Kerlone	Cardioselective BB	Betaxolol HCl 10+, 20 tablets
Lebetol HCl injection	Noncardioselective BB and α_1–blocker	Lebetalol HCl 5/mL IV
Labetalol HCl tablets	Noncardioselective BB and α_1–blocker	Labetalol HCl 100+, 200+, 300+ tablets
Lasix	Diuretic loop	Furosemide 20, 40+, 80 tablets
Levatol	Noncardioselective BB	Penbutolol sulfate 20+ tablets
Lopressor	Cardioselective BB	Metoprolol tartrate 50+, 100+ tablets

(continued on next page)

Table 6
(continued)

Name	Class	Dose Available (mg)
Lopressor HCT	Cardioselective BB and diuretic	Metoprolol tartrate/HCTZ 50/25+, 100/25+, 100/50+ tablets
Lotensin	ACEI	Benazepril HCl 5, 10, 20, 40 tablets
Lotensin HCT	ACEI and diuretic	Benazepril HCl/HCTZ 5/6.25+, 10/12.5+, 20/12.5+, 20/25+ tablets
Lotrel	CCB dihydropyridine and ACEI	Amlodipine besylate/benazepril 2.5/10, 5/10, 5/20, 5/20, 5/40, 10/20, 10/40 caps
Mavik	ACEI	Trandolapril 1+, 2, 4, tablets
Maxide	Diuretic combination	Triamterene/HCTZ 75/50+
Maxzide 25 mg	Diuretic combination	Triamterene/HCTZ 37.5/25+ tablets
Methyldopa	Central α-agonist	Methyldopa 125, 250, 500 tablets
Micardis	ARB	Telmisartan 20, 40, 80 tablets
Micardis HCT	ARB and diuretic	Telmisartan/HCTZ 40/12.5, 80/12.5, 80/25 tablets
Microzide	Diuretic	HCTZ 12.5 caps
Minipress	α$_1$-blocker quinazoline	Prazosin HCl 1, 2, 5 caps
Minoxidil	Vasodilator	Minoxidil 2.5+, 10+ tablets
Nexiclon XR	Central α-agonist	Clonidine 0.17, 0.26, ext-rel tablets
Nexiclon XR oral suspension	Central α-agonist	Clonidine 0.09/mL ext-rel oral susp
Nicardipine	CCB dihydropyridine	Nicardipine HCl 20, 30 caps
Nitropress	Vasodilator	Sodium nitroprusside 25/mL IV
Norvasc	CCB dihydropyridine	Amlodipine as besylate 2.5, 5, 10 tablets
Phentolamine	α-Adrenergic blocker	Phentolamine mesylate 5/vial IM or IV
Pindolol	Noncardioselective BB	Pindolol 5, 10 tablets
Plendil	CCB dihydropyridine	Felodipine 2.5, 5, 10 ext-rel tablets
Prinivila	ACEI	Lisinopril 2.5, 5+, 10, 20, 40 tablets

(continued on next page)

Table 6
(continued)

Name	Class	Dose Available (mg)
Prinzide	ACEI and diuretic	Lisinopril/HCTZ 10/12.5, 20/12.5, 20/25 tablets
Procardia XL	CCB dihydropyridine	Nifedipine 30, 60, 90 ext-rel tablets
Reserpine	Rauwolfia compound	Reserpine 0.1, 0.25 tablets
Sectral	Cardioselective BB	Acebutolol HCl 200, 400 caps
Sular	CCB dihydropyridine	Nisoldipine 8.5, 17, 25.5, 34, ext-rel tablets
Tarka	ACEI and CCB diphenylalkylamine	Trandolapril/verapamil HCl 2/180, 1/240, 2/240, 4/240 ext-rel tablets
Tekamlo	Renin inhibitor and CCB dihydropyridine	Aliskiren/amlodipine 150/5, 150/10, 300/5, 300/5, 300/10 tablets
Tekturna	Direct rennin inhibitor	Aliskiren 150, 300 tablets
Tekturna HCT	Direct rennin inhibitor and diuretic	Aliskiren/HCTZ 150/12.5, 150/25, 300/12.5, 300/25 tablets
Tenex	Central α2-agonist	Guanfacine as HCl 1, 2 tablets
Tenoretic 100	Cardioselective BB and diuretic	Atenolol/chlorthalidone 100/25 tablets
Tenoretic 50	Cardioselective BB and diuretic	Atenolol/chlorthalidone 50/25+ tablets
Tenormin	Cardioselective BB	Atenolol 25, 50, 100 tablets
Teveten	ARB	Eprosartan as mesylate 400, 600 tablets
Teveten HCT	ARB and diuretic	Eprosartan as mesylate/HCTZ 600/12.5, 600/25 tablets
Thalitone	Diuretic monosulfamyl	Chlorthalidone 15 tablets
Tiazac	CCB benzothiazepine	Diltiazem HCl 120, 180, 240, 300, 360, 420 ext-rel beads in caps
Timolol maleate	Noncardioselective BB	Timolol maleate 5, 10+, 20+ tablets
Toprol XL	Cardioselective BB	Metolprolol succinate 25+, 50+, 100+, 200+ ext-rel tablets
Trandate	Noncardioselective BB and α1-blocker	Labetalol HCl 100+, 200+ tablets

(continued on next page)

Table 6
(continued)

Name	Class	Dose Available (mg)
Tribenzor	ARB, dihydropyridine CCB, and thiazide diuretic	Olmesartan medoxomil/amlodipine besylate/HCTZ 20/5/12.5, 40/5/12.5, 40/5/25, 40/10/12.5, 40/10/25 tablets
Twynsta	ARB and CCB	Telmisartan/amlodipine 40/5, 40/10, 80/5, 80/10 tablets
Uniretic	ACEI and diuretic	Moexipril HCl/HCTZ 7.5/12.5+, 15/12.5+, 15/25+ tablets
Univasc	ACEI	Moexipril HCl 7.5+, 15+ tablets
Valturna	Direct rennin inhibitor and ARB	Aliskiren/valsartan 150/160, 300/320 tablets
Vaseretic	ACEI and diuretic	Enalapril maleate/HCTZ 10/25 tablets
Vasotec	ACEI	Enalapril maleate 2.5+, 5+, 10+, 20+ tablets
Verelan	CCB diphenylalkylamine	Verapamil HCl 120, 180, 240, 360 sus-rel caps
Verelan PM	CCB diphenylalkylamine	Verapamil HCl 100, 200, 300 controlled-onset ext-rel caps
Zaroxoyn	Diuretic quinazoline	Metolazone 2.5, 5, 10 tablets
Zebeta	Cardioselective BB	Bisoprolol fumarate 5+, 10 tablets
Zestoretic	ACEI and diuretic	Lisinopril/HCTZ 10/12.5, 20/12.5, 20/25 tablets
Zestril	ACEI	Lisinopril 2.5, 5, 10, 20, 30, 40 tablets
Ziac	Cardioselective BB and diuretic	Bisoprolol fumarate/HCTZ 2.5/6.25, 5/6.25, 10/6.25 tablets

+, Scored tablet.
Abbreviations: cap, capsule; ext-rel, extended release; HCTZ, hydrochlorothiazide; HMG-CoA reductase, 3-hydroxy-3-methyl-glutaryl-CoA reductase; IM, intramuscular; IV, intravenous; K+, potassium; sus-re, sustained release; susp, suspension.

Diuretics

Thiazide diuretics, the most commonly used type of diuretic, inhibit the sodium chloride transporter in the distal tubule. The sodium chloride transporter only reabsorbs about 5% of the filtered sodium and therefore is less efficacious than loop diuretics in producing diuresis and natriuresis. Because thiazide diuretics increase sodium delivery to the distal segment of the distal tubule, potassium is lost and hypokalemia may occur. Adverse effects include electrolyte disorders, hyperglycemia, hyperuricemia, photosensitivity, orthostatic hypotension, gastrointestinal disturbances, and adverse lipid profile. Use caution in the elderly and patients with renal impairment, hepatic impairment, arrhythmias, diabetes, asthma, systemic lupus, postsympathectomy, and excessive fluid loss. Contraindications include anuria and sulfonamide allergy. Thiazide diuretics are pregnancy category C. Breast-feeding is not recommended.

Loop diuretics inhibit the sodium-potassium-chloride cotransporter in the distal tubule. This transporter normally reabsorbs about 25% of the sodium load and causes inhibition of this pump leading to a significant increase in the distal tubular concentration of sodium, reduced hypertonicity of the surrounding interstitium, and less water reabsorption in the collecting duct. Like thiazide diuretics, loop diuretics cause diuresis and natriuresis. This class also induces renal synthesis of prostaglandins, which contributes to their renal action including the increase in renal blood flow and redistribution of renal cortical blood flow. Common reactions include urinary frequency, dizziness, nausea, vomiting, weakness, muscle cramps, hypokalemia, hypomagnesemia, orthostatic hypotension, increased alanineaminotransferase, increased aspartate aminotransferase, blurred vision, anorexia, abdominal cramps, diarrhea, pruritus, rash, hyperuricemia, hyperglycemia, hypocalcemia, tinnitus, paresthesias, photosensitivity, increased cholesterol, and increase in triglycerides. Contraindications include hypersensitivity to the drug class, anuria, hepatic coma, and electrolyte imbalances. Precautions include diabetes mellitus, acute myocardial infarction, arrhythmias, hearing impairment, concurrent ototoxic agents, systemic lupus, hepatic impairment, severe renal disease, urinary retention, pancreatitis, hypertension during pregnancy, premature neonates, elderly patients, and use with iodinated contrast.

Potassium-sparing diuretics do not act directly on sodium transport. Some of the drugs in this class antagonize the actions of aldosterone at the distal segment of the distal tubule and are referred to as aldosterone receptor antagonists. Aldosterone receptor antagonists cause sodium to pass into the collecting duct and be excreted in urine. They are potassium sparing because inhibition of aldosterone-sensitive sodium reabsorption causes less potassium and hydrogen ion exchange for sodium by this transporter. Other potassium-sparing diuretics directly inhibit sodium channels associated with the aldosterone-sensitive sodium, and therefore have similar effects on sodium and hydrogen ions as the aldosterone antagonists. This class of diuretic is weak and is often combined with thiazide and loop diuretics to help prevent hypokalemia. Common adverse side effects include hyperkalemia, metabolic alkalosis, hypomagnesemia, hyperuricemia, dehydration, and dose-related hearing loss. Contraindications include hypersensitivity to the drug class, hyperkalemia, and anuria. Precautions include renal impairment, creatinine greater than 1.5 mg/dL, diabetic nephropathy, and diabetes mellitus.

Calcium Channel Blockers

Calcium channel blockers bind to L-type calcium channels located on the vascular smooth muscle, cardiac myocytes, and cardiac nodal tissue, which regulate the influx of calcium into muscle cells, stimulating smooth muscle contraction and cardiac myocyte contraction. By blocking calcium entry into the cell, calcium channel blockers cause vascular smooth muscle relaxation, decreased myocardial force generation, decreased heart rate, and decreased conduction velocity within the heart, especially in the atrioventricular node. Calcium channel blockers reduce arterial blood pressure by decreasing systemic vascular resistance.

There are 3 classes of calcium channel blockers. The dihydropyridines reduce systemic vascular resistance and arterial pressure and are primarily used in the treatment of hypertension. Common adverse side effects of dihydropyridines include peripheral edema, headache, fatigue, palpitations, dizziness, nausea, and flushing. Contraindications include hypersensitivity to the drug class. Precautions include severe coronary artery disease, severe aortic stenosis, congestive heart failure, severe hepatic impairment, and elderly patients.

The nondihydropyridines class contains only 2 drugs: verapamil and diltiazem. Verapamil is in the phenylalkylamine class, is selective for the myocardium, and is less effective as a systemic vasodilator drug. Diltiazem is a benzophiazepine and is intermediate between verapamil and dihydropyridines in its selectivity for vascular calcium channels and is therefore able to reduce arterial pressure without producing the same degree of reflex cardiac stimulation as is caused by dihydropyridines. Common adverse side effects of nondihydropyridines include peripheral edema, headache, dizziness, flushing, fatigue, weakness, nausea, constipation, muscle cramps, nervousness, palpitations, dyspnea, nasal congestion, and hypotension. Contraindications of the nondihydropyridines include hypersensitivity to the drug class, lactose intolerance, and hypertensive crisis. Precautions include congestive heart failure, aortic stenosis, hypertension, renal impairment, hepatic impairment, anesthesia, surgery, concurrent or recent use of a BB, severe gastrointestinal stricture, gastrointestinal hypomotility disorder, and in the elderly patient.

BBs

BBs bind to β-adrenoceptors and block the binding of norepinephrine and epinephrine to these receptors, which inhibits normal sympathetic effects that act through these receptors. The partial agonist BBs are sympatholytic drugs that partially activate the receptor while preventing norepinephrine from binding to the receptor. They possess intrinsic sympathomimetic activity. Some BBs possess membrane-stabilizing activity. The first-generation BBs are nonselective and possess both β1 and β2 adrenoreceptors. Second-generation BBs are more cardioselective because they are selective for β1 adrenoreceptors. The relative selectivity can be lost at higher drug dosages. The third-generation BBs possess vasodilator actions through blockade of vascular α-adrenoreceptors. BBs decrease arterial blood pressure by reducing cardiac output. A BB should not be used for acute treatment of hypertension because it is not effective in reducing arterial pressure because of a compensatory increase in systemic vascular resistance. This class also inhibits the release of renin by the kidney, which decreases angiotensin II and aldosterone. Common adverse effects include bradycardia, reduced exercise capacity, heart failure, hypertension, atrioventricular nodal conduction block, bronchoconstriction, and decreased awareness of hypoglycemia. Contraindications include sinus bradycardia and partial atrioventricular block. Precautions include concomitant use with cardioselective calcium channel blockers such as verapamil because of their additive effects in producing electrical and mechanical depression.

α-Adrenoceptor Antagonists (α-Blockers)

α-Adrenoceptor antagonists (α-blockers) block the effect of sympathetic nerves on blood vessels by binding to α-adrenoreceptors located on the vascular smooth muscle and compete antagonistically to the binding of norepinephrine that is released by sympathetic nerves synapsing on smooth muscle. Vascular smooth muscle has 2 primary types of α-adrenoceptors: α_1 and α_2. The α_1-adrenoceptors are located on the vascular smooth muscle; the α_2-adrenoceptors are located on the sympathetic nerve terminals and on the vascular smooth muscle. α_1-adrenoceptors antagonists cause vasodilatation by blocking the binding of norepinephrine to the smooth muscle receptors. α-Blockers dilate both arteries and veins because both vessel types are innervated by sympathetic adrenergic nerves; the vasodilator effect is more pronounced in the arterial resistance vessels. The newer α-blockers on the market are selective antagonists compared with the older drugs, which are nonselective antagonists. Common side effects include dizziness, orthostatic hypotension, nasal congestion, headache, fluid retention, and reflex tachycardia.

Centrally Acting Sympatholytics

Centrally acting sympatholytics block the sympathetic adrenergic system at 3 different levels. Peripheral sympatholytic drugs include α-adrenoreceptors and β-adrenoreceptor antagonists. They block the effects of norepinephrine at the heart and blood vessels. Ganglionic blockers block the impulse transmission at the sympathetic ganglia. Centrally acting sympatholytics block sympathetic activity within the brain. This class is not considered to be first-line therapy in the treatment of hypertension. It is generally used in conjunction with a diuretic to prevent fluid accumulation. Medications in this class include clonidine, guanabenz, guanfacine, and methyldopa. Common side effects include sedation, dry mouth, dry nasal mucosa, bradycardia, orthostatic hypotension, impotence, constipation, nausea, gastric upset, fluid retention, and edema. Discontinuation of clonidine can lead to rebound hypertension.

Direct-acting Vasodilators

The direct-acting vasodilator class has only 1 drug: hydralazine. Hydralazine's mechanism of action is not clear; it seems to have direct effects on vascular smooth muscle. It causes smooth muscle hyperpolarization through the opening of potassium channels and inhibits IP_3-induced release of calcium from smooth muscle sarcoplasmic reticulum, and stimulates the formation of nitric oxide by the vascular endothelium, leading to cGMP-mediated vasodilation, which leads to a reduced systemic vascular resistance and arterial pressure. It is not generally used as monotherapy. It is not first-line therapy. It has a short half-life, which necessitates frequent dosing. It can cause reflex tachycardia, which makes it undesirable for treating chronic hypertension. It is used to treat acute hypertension emergencies. It is often used in conjunction with a BB and diuretic to reduce the risk of reflex tachycardia. Common side effects include headaches, flushing, and tachycardia.

Nitrodilators

Nitrodilators include 2 basic types: one that releases nitric oxide spontaneously and organic nitrates that require an enzymatic process to form nitric oxide. Nitric oxide activates smooth muscle soluble guanylyl cyclase to form cGMP. Increased intracellular cGMP inhibits calcium entry into the cell. Decreased intracellular calcium concentrations cause smooth muscle relaxation. Nitrodilators cause vasodilation, decreased venous pressure, and decreased arterial pressure. This class is not used to treat chronic primary or secondary hypertension. It is used to treat acute hypertensive emergencies from conditions such as the pheochromocytoma, renal artery stenosis, and aortic dissection. Common side effects include headache, cutaneous flushing, postural hypotension, and reflex tachycardia.

Potassium Channel Openers

Potassium channel openers open ATP-sensitive potassium channels in vascular smooth muscle causing voltage-gated calcium channels to decrease intracellular calcium. Decreased intracellular calcium causes relaxation and vasodilation, decreased systemic vascular resistance, and decreased arterial pressure. There is only 1 drug in this class: minoxidial. It is not used as first-line therapy for hypertension because of side effects. It is commonly used in conjunction with BBs and diuretics. Common side effects include headaches, flushing, and reflex tachycardia.

Renin Inhibitors

Renin inhibitors affect the renin-angiotensin-aldosterone system. Renin inhibitors inhibit the activity of renin preventing angiotensin II formation and producing vasodilation. Renin is produced by the kidney in response to sympathetic activation, hypertension, and decreased sodium delivery to the distal renal tubule. Renin causes angiotensinogen to form angiotensin I. Angiotensin I is converted to angiotensin II by ACE. Angiotensin II causes vasoconstriction, stimulation of aldosterone, renal retention of sodium and water, and increased sympathetic activity, and it stimulates cardiac and vascular hypertrophy. Renin inhibitors dilate arteries and veins, downregulate sympathetic adrenergic activity, promote renal excretion of sodium and water, and inhibit cardiac and vascular remodeling. Renin inhibitors are generally well tolerated. The incidence of cough is lower than in patients who take an ACEI. Angioedema is possible but rare. Diarrhea is observed in less than 3% of the patients. If taken with an ACEI, hyperkalemia may occur, especially in patients with diabetes. There is no additional benefit to combining a renin inhibitor with an ACEI or ARB in patients with diabetes. Renin inhibitors cannot be used during pregnancy.

SUMMARY

Hypertension management in patients with diabetes is important for the reduction of risk for microvascular and macrovascular complications of diabetes. Many trials have been conducted in regard to goals for blood pressure in patients with diabetes and the best drugs to use. National organizations such as the American diabetes Association, and US Department of Health and Human Resources have published guidelines for the management of hypertension in patients with diabetes. It is important to understand how antihypertensive medications work, their common side effects, and how to use them in combination to achieve pressure targets.

REFERENCES

1. American Diabetes Association. Standards of medical care in diabetes-2012. Diabetes Care 2012;35(Suppl 1):S11–63.
2. Turner RC, Holman RR, Matthews DR. Hypertension in Diabetes Study (HDS): prevalence of hypertension in newly presenting type 2 diabetic patients and the association with risk factors for cardiovascular and diabetic complications. J Hypertens 1993;11:309–17.
3. Arauz-Pacheco C, Parrott M, Raskin P. Treatment of hypertension in adult patients with diabetes. Diabetes Care 2002;25:134–47.
4. Sowers JR, Epstein M, Frohlich ED. Diabetes, hypertension, and cardiovascular disease: an update. Hypertension 2001;37:1053–9.
5. Parving HH, Hommel E, Mathiesen E. Prevalence of micro albumin area, arterial hypertension, retinopathy and neuropathy in patients with insulin-dependent diabetes. Br Med J (Clin Res Ed) 1988;96:156.
6. Mogensen EE, Hansen KW, Petersen MM. Renal factors influencing blood pressure threshold and choice of treatment for hypertension in IDDM. Diabetes Care 1991;14:13.
7. Cruickshank K, Riste L, Anderson SG. The aortic pulse-wave velocity and its relationship mortality in diabetes and glucose intolerance: an integrated index of vascular function? Circulation 2002;106:2085.
8. The ACCORD Study Group. Effects of intensive blood pressure control in type 2 diabetes mellitus. N Engl J Med 2010;362:1575–85.

9. ADVANCE Collaborative Group. Effects of a fixed combination of perindopril and indapamide on macrovascular and microvascular outcomes in patients with type 2 diabetes mellitus (the ADVANCE trial): a randomized controlled trial. Lancet 2007;370:829–40.
10. Pepine C, Handberg E, Cooper-DeHoff R. A calcium antagonists vs a non-calcium antagonist hypertension treatment strategy for patients with coronary artery disease: the International Verapamil-Trandolapril study (INVEST): a randomized controlled trial. JAMA 2003;290:2805–16.
11. United States Department of Health and Human Services. The seventh report of the Joint National Committee on Prevention, Detection, Evaluation, and Treatment of High Blood Pressure. August 2004. Available at: www.nhlbi.hih.gov. Accessed September 29, 2012.
12. Bakris G, Sarafidis PA, Weir M. Renal outcomes with different fixed-dose combination therapies in patients with hypertension at high risk for cardiovascular events (ACCO MPL ISH) a pre-specified secondary analysis of a randomized controlled trial. Lancet 2010;375:1173–81.

Diabetes and Heart Failure

Talar L. Glover, MS, RN, CNS, CDE[a],*,
Esperanza Galvan, MS, RN, CVRN, CDE[b]

KEYWORDS

- Heart failure • Diabetes • Diabetes complications

KEY POINTS

- Heart failure affects over 5 million Americans and is a health and financial burden to the US health care system.
- The 5-year mortality of heart failure with diabetes is about 50%.
- Health care providers should be aware of the Joint Commission Core Measures for treating patients with heart failure.

HEART FAILURE FACTS

Heart failure affects over five million Americans. It is a common condition affecting the older adult population. As life expectancy increases, heart failure will become more of a health and financial burden to the US health care system. There are 550,000 new cases diagnosed each year.[1] The 5-year mortality of heart failure with diabetes is about 50%. Seventy five percent of patients with heart failure have hypertension. Eighty percent of admissions arrive through the emergency department. Heart failure is the most costly reason for admission of patients over 65 years of age. The Joint Commission has developed core measures for heart failure treatment. See **Box 1**. For the hospitalized patient to have the best outcome it is recommended that communication improve between physicians and nurses, that a process is in place for seamless transitions between care settings, that there is medication reconciliation, and that clear consistent documentation is in place for every heart failure patient at discharge from the hospital.[2] Other measures to consider for monitoring include: readmission for heart failure, length of stay, discharge on beta blocker, and vaccination rate.

Heart failure results from any disorder of the heart that alters the ventricle's ability to fill and eject blood. The heart becomes incapable of sustaining a cardiac output sufficient to meet metabolic requirements and cope with venous return. Signs and symptoms are related to a change in ventricular and valvular function and response

The authors have nothing to disclose.
[a] Diabetes Service Line and Patient Education, Harris Health System, 2525 Holly Hall Street, Houston, TX 77054, USA; [b] CardioPulmonary Management Program, Harris Health System, 2525 Holly Hall Street, Houston, TX 77054, USA
* Corresponding author.
E-mail address: talar.glover@harrishealth.org

Box 1
The Joint Commission Core Measures for Heart Failure

- Discharge on angiotensin-converting enzyme inhibitor
- Smoking cessation counseling
- Heart failure discharge instructions
  - Definition of heart failure
  - Lifestyle: nutrition, fluids, activity
  - Medications
  - Warning signs
  - When to get help
  - Follow-up care
- Left ventricular ejection fraction assessment

Data from The Joint Commission Core Measures for Heart Failure. 2012. Available at: www.jointcommission.org/core_measure_sets.aspx. Accessed October 1, 2012.

---

to load conditions.[3] With systolic heart failure, the left ventricle contracts abnormally and, with diastolic heart failure, the left ventricle does not relax normally. Right-sided heart failure usually results from left-sided failure. Causes of heart failure are listed in **Box 2**.

Box 2
Causes of heart failure

Coronary artery disease

Myocardial infarction

Left ventricular systolic dysfunction

Hypertension

Hyperthyroidism

Alcohol use

Abnormal heart valves

Congenital defects

Severe lung disease

Arrhythmias or dysrhythmias

Severe anemia

Myocarditis

Cardiomyopathy

Obesity

Diabetes

Data from Tracy CM, Epstein AE, Darbar D, et al. 2012 ACCF/AHA/HRS focused update of the 2008 guidelines for device-based therapy of cardiac rhythm abnormalities: a report of the American College of Cardiology Foundation/American Heart Association Task Force on Practice Guidelines. Circulation 2012;126:1784–800.

Diabetes contributes to the development of heart failure in many ways, including

- Dyslipidemia, which may lead to hypertension, coronary heart disease, and myocardial infarction
- Hyperglycemia, which may lead to electrolyte imbalance, arrhythmia, or dysrhythmia
- Autonomic neuropathy, which may lead to cardiomyopathy with impaired left ventricular function, higher workload, resting tachycardia, and postural hypotension
- Diabetes medications (eg, thiazolidinediones), which can increase vascular volume
- Renal failure, which can lead to electrolyte imbalance and fluid retention.

There are three types of cardiomyopathy:

- Dilated (congestive): muscle fibers are damaged resulting in dilation of heart chambers
- Hypertrophic (idiopathic hypertrophic subaortic stenosis [IHSS]): asymmetric thickening of the septum with left ventricular hypertrophy and diastolic dysfunction
- Restrictive: fibrosis and thickening of the endocardium, which restricts filling of the ventricles.

All three types of cardiomyopathy have been associated with diabetes.

DIAGNOSTIC TOOLS

Diagnostic tools have advanced beyond chest radiographs and ECGs. Laboratory and radiographic findings, and an assessment of functional capacity, assist in developing a definitive diagnosis. The B-type natriuretic peptide (BNP) can be used as a reliable diagnostic tool for heart failure because it can differentiate pulmonary and cardiac dyspnea, correlate with excess intravascular volume, and reliably detect left ventricular dysfunction.[4] However, the most useful test continues to be the echocardiogram, which can distinguish between systolic and diastolic dysfunction. See **Box 3** for diagnostic tests.

Box 3
Diagnostic tests for heart failure

Chest radiograph

ECG

Exercise stress test

Complete blood cell count (CBC)

Liver function tests

Serum urea nitrogen or creatinine (BUN)

B-type natriuretic peptide (BNP)

Echocardiography to determine ejection fraction

Cardiac MRI

Cardiac catheterization

Angiography

Radionuclide ventriculography or multiple gated acquisition scan (MUGA)

ASSESSMENT

Patient history can assist with effective treatment and education as well as determine the progression of heart failure. Subjective reports may include weight gain, edema, fatigue, dyspnea, orthopnea, paroxysmal nocturnal dyspnea, nonproductive cough or hemoptysis, chest pain, dizziness, lightheadedness, confusion, exercise intolerance, and poor appetite. Medical history of hypertension, diabetes, myocardial infarction, or renal failure should raise suspicion. Medication review will often show multiple drugs for the management of hypertension or fluid retention, rhythm stabilizers, and vasodilators (**Table 1** includes the most common drugs used in heart failure).

Physical examination may reveal tachycardia, S3, an extra heart sound that occurs after the normal two heart sounds, is an early sign; hypotension; narrow pulse pressure; jugular-venous distension; abdominal, peripheral, pretibial, or periorbital edema; lung crackles; shortness of breath or labored breathing before or while speaking; and cool extremities.

TREATMENT

Treatment is based on the stage of heart failure. The American College of Cardiology Foundation and the American Heart Association have set practice guidelines to support health care providers in clinical decision-making when managing the heart failure patient.[1] It is up to the health care provider and the patient to work collaboratively and decide on the treatment plan that offers the highest quality of care and quality of life to the patient (**Table 2**). Before the development of symptoms, treatment is focused on lifestyle change and medications that will decrease risk factors to prevent damage to the heart. After symptoms develop, medications are added to decrease workload and slow progression to the next stage.

Table 1
Common heart failure drugs

Drug Type	Actions	Cautions
ACE inhibitor	• Control blood pressure • Allow vasodilation • Reduce oxidative stress	• Monitor potassium • Angioedema • Cough
ARB	• Control blood pressure • Allow vasodilation • Reduce oxidative stress	• Monitor potassium • Angioedema
Diuretic	• Control blood pressure • Decrease intravascular volume • Reduce fluid retention	• Monitor potassium • Hyperglycemia
Digoxin	• Cardiotonic • Reduce arrhythmia	• Monitor potassium • Bradycardia • Doses at least 12 h apart
Beta blocker	• Slow heart rate • Reduce arrhythmia • Decrease contractility and workload	• Hypotension • Bradycardia • Edema
Spironolactone	• Control blood pressure • Reduce potassium loss	• Monitor potassium • Arrhythmias • Breast swelling
Vasodilators	• Control blood pressure • Vasodilation	• Postural hypotension

Abbreviations: ACE, angiotensin-converting enzyme; ARB, angiotensin receptor blocker.

Table 2
Classifications of heart failure

NYHA Functional Classification	Stages of Heart Failure (American Heart Association)	Treatment Recommendations
I Normal, no symptoms with activities of daily living	A Has established risk factors for development but no cardiac structural disorder and is asymptomatic	Treat risk factors to slow disease progress • Hypertension ACE or ARB • Lipids • Stop smoking • Exercise • Limit or stop alcohol • Control metabolic syndrome or diabetes
II Normal activities cause symptoms, relieved with rest	B Has cardiac structural disorder, but is asymptomatic	Continue lifestyle changes • ACE or ARB • Beta blockers in some • Implantable defibrillator if needed
III Minimal activity causes symptoms, no symptoms at rest	C Has past or present heart failure symptoms associated with cardiac structural disorder	Add sodium restriction to lifestyle • ACE or ARB • Diuretics • Beta blockers In selected patients • Aldosterone antagonist • Digitalis • Hydralazine or nitrates Devices if needed • Implantable defibrillator • Biventricular pacing
IV Symptomatic at rest	D Has refractory (end-stage) heart failure and requires specialized care	Consider end-of-life care • Heart transplant in some patients

Abbreviations: ACE, angiotensin-converting enzyme; ARB, angiotensin receptor blocker; NYHA, New York Heart Association.
Data from Lindenfeld J, Albert NM, Boehmer JP, et al. Executive summary: HFSA 2010 comprehensive heart failure practice guideline. J Card Fail 2010;16:475–539.

Surgical procedures used to treat heart failure aim to increase blood flow to the ailing heart. These include transmyocardial revascularization, resynchronization of the ventricles (biventricular pacing), or decreasing the size of the ventricle (Dor procedure). At stage D, some patients may be evaluated for mechanical circulatory support. Devices such as left ventricular assist devices may be used while waiting for cardiac transplantation.[5] If transplant is not an option, palliative or hospice care may be the only choice.

INPATIENT MANAGEMENT

The principles of inpatient management of heart failure are

- Rapid diagnosis: determine cause of symptoms or exacerbation
  - BNP
  - Cardiovascular-related: myocardial infarction, arrhythmia, hypertension, pulmonary embolus
  - Infection
  - Renal failure
  - Medical or dietary nonadherence
- Oxygen therapy: pulse oximetry
- Monitoring
  - Cardiac, including ECG, central pressures if available, vital signs
  - Intake and output
  - Daily weight
  - Clinical signs of perfusion and congestion
- Intravenous (IV) fluids or medications
  - Loop diuretics if significant fluid overload
  - Vasodilators: nitroprusside, nitroglycerin, nesiritide
  - Inotropes: dopamine, dobutamine, milrinone
  - Thromboembolic prophylaxis
  - IV fluids limited.

Control of blood glucose can decrease length of stay. The routine treatment of hyperglycemia is often a fluid bolus, which is contraindicated with heart failure. Fluid restriction may make it more difficult to control blood glucose. Initially, an insulin drip may be ordered for hyperglycemia. Hyperglycemia may persist despite insulin infusion. This can signal a catabolic state and potential for lactic acidosis if the patient is not able to eat, increasing the insulin drip rate and adding dextrose infusion is warranted. Remember, a liter of 5% dextrose only contains 200 calories.

Blood glucose monitoring can be a challenge in patients with significant edema. If the bedside meter will accept venous or capillary blood, these alternatives should be considered. However, the blood glucose check may be hourly with an insulin drip, potentially causing anemia if blood has to be wasted.

Drugs that can exacerbate heart failure, such as metformin and the thiazolidinedione, should be discontinued. Secretagogues, such as sulfonylureas and glinides, may be contraindicated if renal function is impaired. Subcutaneous insulin absorption may be affected by edema and poor capillary circulation.

CASE STUDY

Mr Jones has stage C heart failure complicated by type 2 diabetes. He recently had pioglitazone added to his regimen of metformin and glyburide because his hemoglobin A1c was 9.4%. He is admitted to the medical intensive care unit with a BNP of 100 pg/mL (done in the emergency center); a blood glucose of 240 mg/dL; orthopnea; a moist cough with frothy sputum; and 4+ pitting edema of his legs, scrotum, and lower abdomen. His admission orders include Lasix IV and an insulin drip.

Questions

1. What could have precipitated his heart failure exacerbation?
2. What IV fluid rate will be most appropriate?
3. What questions can you ask to assess his self-care and daily activities?
4. What diabetes medicines should he be given at discharge?

SUMMARY

Health care providers must offer the best possible care for the more than five million Americans who experience heart failure and help ease the health and financial burden of these cases on the US health care system. Effective and cost-effective treatment is the standard offered by The Joint Commission Core Measures for Heart Failure and serves as a guide to reaching these goals.

REFERENCES

1. Jessup M, Abraham WT, Casey DE, et al. Writing on behalf of the 2005 Guideline Update for the Diagnosis and Management of Chronic Heart Failure in the Adult Writing Committee. 2009 Focused update: ACCF/AHA guidelines for the diagnosis and management of heart failure in adults: a report of the American College of Cardiology Foundation/American Heart Association Task Force on Practice Guidelines. Circulation 2009;119:1977–2016.
2. Lindenfeld J, Albert NM, Boehmer JP, et al. Executive summary: HFSA 2010 comprehensive heart failure practice guideline. J Card Fail 2010;16:475–539.
3. Tracy CM, Epstein AE, Darbar D, et al. 2012 ACCF/AHA/HRS focused update of the 2008 guidelines for device-based therapy of cardiac rhythm abnormalities: a report of the American College of Cardiology Foundation/American Heart Association Task Force on Practice Guidelines. Circulation 2012;126:1784–800.
4. Aspromonte N, Feola M, Milli M, et al. Prognostic role of B-type natriuretic peptide in patients with diabetes and acute decompensated heart failure. Diabet Med 2007;24(2):124–30.
5. Uriel N, Naka Y, Colombo P, et al. Improved diabetic control in advanced heart failure patients treated with left ventricular assist devices. Eur J Heart Fail 2011; 13(2):195–9. http://dx.doi.org/10.1093/eurjhf/hfq204.

Diabetes Education in Hospitalized Children
Developmental and Situational Concerns

Barb Schreiner, PhD, RN, CDE, BC-ADM, CPLP

KEYWORDS

- PICU • Children • Type 1 diabetes • Diabetes self-management education
- Hospitalization

KEY POINTS

- The family of a child newly diagnosed with diabetes in the pediatric intensive care unit requires intensive survival skills education and emotional support.
- Critical care nurses play a vital role in assisting the patient and family with coping and learning diabetes self-care skills.
- Critical care nurses need to learn current diabetes survival skills to assist the patient and family in acquiring all the necessary diabetes self-management skills.

Jack is a bright, energetic, 6-year-old boy who has been admitted to the pediatric intensive care unit (PICU) in diabetic ketoacidosis (DKA) resulting from his newly diagnosed type 1 diabetes (T1DM). Jack is somnolent with a blood glucose (BG) level of 514 mg/dL and pH of 7.25. His treatment team has initiated intravenous fluids and an insulin drip. Jack's parents are distraught and in shock. They are frightened by the PICU environment and unsure of what to do next. They blame themselves for not catching the symptoms earlier. Jack's father has a relative with type 2 diabetes (T2DM) but no one in the family has T1DM. Jack's mother is a schoolteacher and his father is a sales representative. His father's job takes him away from home several days a week. Jack has a 9-year-old sister who is anxious about Jack and is presently staying with her maternal grandparents near home. Is it time to begin diabetes education with this family?

Janequa is 14 years old and has been readmitted to the PICU for the second time this year in DKA. Janequa has had T1DM for 6 years, has been to diabetes camp 3 times, and started using a continuous insulin infusion pump 2 years ago. She lives with her mother, an attorney, her father, a chef and restaurant owner, and 2 healthy

Department of Nursing, Capella University, 225 South Sixth Street, 9th Floor, Minneapolis, MN 55402, USA
E-mail address: barb.schreiner@sbcglobal.net

siblings. Janequa routinely visits her diabetes team, including an endocrinologist, a team psychologist, dietitian, and diabetes nurse. For the first few years of her diabetes, her hemoglobin A1c (HbA1c) ranged from 7.7% to 8.7% indicating an average BG of 170 to 190 mg/dL. But more recently, her diabetes control has slipped. Her HbA1c is presently 10.1% (estimated average BG of 240 mg/dL). A review of her pump memory indicates that she has missed several meal doses and she did not make the basal rate adjustments recommended by her team. Janequa is a good student, typically making the honor roll in her classes. She is active in cheerleading and volleyball. Is this the right time to provide a refresher course in diabetes?

Gone are the days of prolonged hospitalizations for the child or adolescent newly diagnosed with diabetes.[1] BG levels are stabilized, acidosis is corrected, and families are discharged in mere days. There is little time to provide the survival skills and education, much less support the family through the impact of the diagnosis. Yet, critical care nurses are in an important position to begin the family's adaptation and recovery. This article explores the educational and support needs of not only the newly diagnosed child but also the child who is repeatedly admitted to the PICU. The role of the critical care nurse is emphasized and tips for returning the family to health are offered.

EDUCATIONAL NEEDS OF THE FAMILY AND CHILD WITH NEWLY DIAGNOSED DIABETES

The onset of T1DM signals a disruption in family life and gradual establishment of new roles, tasks, and relationships. Not only does the child need to adjust to changes in diet and invasive tests and therapies, but they must also deal with their parents' response to the diagnosis. Even very young children can detect a parent's anxiety. School-aged children quickly latch onto a teacher's concern or a school nurse's over-concern. For some children, this quickly becomes a source of manipulation. So what can a critical care nurse do to help a family begin their diabetes journey feeling supported?

In the initial days of managing diabetes, families have 5 basic survival needs: safety, simple pathophysiology, skills, school, and support. These 5 Ss, provided when the family is ready, are critical to early success with diabetes. **Table 1** provides an overview of the critical care nurse's role in each of the 5 Ss.

Table 1 Diabetes education and the role of the critical care nurse	
Topic	**Critical Care Nurse's Role**
Safety	Check adequacy of literacy and numeracy skills Teach about the symptoms and treatment of hypoglycemia Identify key times to call for help
Simple pathophysiology	Provide simple clear explanations Deliver education with hope and confidence
Skills	Pair procedures with matter-of-fact health messages Encourage parent participation in BG checks and insulin injections
School	Offer resources to help families return child to school Suggest ways to prepare school staff for the child's safe return
Support	Assess adequacy of parents' support network Suggest resources to support parents Provide the child with developmentally appropriate support Remember sibling needs

SAFETY

Parents and older children must understand the danger zones of BG levels. Knowing how to identify hypoglycemia and hyperglycemia are early important skills. Knowing what to do is equally important, even if it only means calling for help with treating or interpreting a BG value.

Surprisingly, many people lack the health literacy and numeracy skills to differentiate the meaning of numbers. For example, if an individual is weak in number sequencing, they cannot decide if 170 is higher or lower than 120. White and colleagues[2] noted that "patients with diabetes and limited health literacy or numeracy are more likely to have poorer disease knowledge and symptom recognition, poorer glycemic control, greater difficulty interpreting food labels and estimating portion sizes, lower self-confidence in diabetes management (ie, self-efficacy), fewer self-management behaviors, and poorer communication with their providers" (p. 238). One of the first strategies to assure safety is to assess how well the child and caregivers understand and use numbers in their daily lives. Several investigators have provided tips for addressing low numeracy skills.[2–4] Using tips such as visuals, adapted BG log books, and modified number scales can help individuals interpret numbers, a critical component to identifying and confirming hypoglycemia.

After assessing and addressing numeracy, parents should be instructed in the symptoms and BG levels associated with hypoglycemia. For parents of very young children, distinguishing hypoglycemia from usual child behavior can be daunting. Is the temper tantrum indicating a low BG level or is it the terrible 2s? Knowing that checking BG can help differentiate behaviors is comforting to parents. Parents are not the only caregivers who must have safety skills. Anyone who supervises the child must be trained in simple approaches to identifying and treating hypoglycemia; this includes grandparents, babysitters, coaches, teachers, school nurses, and others. Parents should leave the hospital with a plan to share important information with others.

SIMPLE PATHOPHYSIOLOGY

Although safety is paramount, a cursory understanding of what goes wrong in diabetes can be reassuring for parents. Much of a parent's initial response to the diagnosis is based on feelings of guilt and confusion.[5] Did they cause the disease? How did it happen? Providing simple clear explanations of the nature and management of T1DM is helpful for parents. At diagnosis, a parent may not be able to fully absorb detailed information, but they remember how the message was delivered and the hope and confidence that was expressed.

SKILLS

Managing diabetes, particularly T1DM, depends on a series of skills and tasks. BG monitoring and insulin injections are 2 of the most important tasks. Emotions surrounding these skills range from quiet acquiescence to outright fear or anger. For most children, these tasks are best done in a straightforward manner. Adding a phrase, "this is your medicine to make your body feel better" or "this quick check will tell us how your body is using food" can link the uncomfortable procedure to a matter-of-fact message about health.

For parents, engaging them early in the skills is essential in building their competence and confidence. Even in the PICU, encouraging parents to care for their child in small but meaningful ways is effective because it restores the parents' role and alleviates some anxiety.[6] Parents should be encouraged to use a BG meter and to prepare and give insulin injections in the supportive environment of the PICU.

SCHOOL

One of the many worries of a parent with a newly diagnosed child is what will happen after the hospitalization. When should the child return to school? How will we ever prepare the school? The child's treatment plan and diabetes team will determine the appropriate time to return to school. In the meantime, the parents can begin to think about what the school needs to know to safely provide health supervision. One valuable resource for parents is the Safe at School program of the American Diabetes Association accessed at the Web site www.diabetes.org. This program offers tips for developing care plans and school staff training.

Federal disability laws protect children with diabetes in most schools. These laws support parents and school personnel in developing care plans to accommodate diabetes care. Such plans may cover time for snacks or restroom breaks, time for BG checks or premeal insulin injections. The care plan should also clearly define emergency care, such as the need for glucagon injection to treat severe hypoglycemia. Although the PICU stay is not the time to fully develop these plans, parents should be aware that these protections are in place for their child.

SUPPORT

"It's not what they told me about the diagnosis that I remember; it's how they told me." Years later, parents remember the emotion-laden time as they work to regain normalcy and routine.[7] Support can look different to each parent. For some, their health care team provides the most support, particularly at diagnosis and in the first weeks of adjustment. For others, support is found in relatives or friends, in their church family or in online social networks. Some parents report that tapping into their humor, faith, optimism, patience, and inner strength helped the most in the early days and later.[8]

The PICU nurse can explore with parents what strategies they have used in the past to deal with upsetting or difficult situations. Simply reminding parents that these same strategies may help now can be reassuring to them. Several online resources are ready to help parents of newly diagnosed children. One of the most credible is the Children With Diabetes network. Started more than 10 years ago by the father of a child with T1DM, this network offers not only online support but regional and national conferences for families with diabetes. The online community may be found at www.childrenwithdiabetes.com.

Community support for parents may also come from local diabetes organizations such as the American Diabetes Association and the Juvenile Diabetes Research Foundation. Both have welcome kits for children and families.

Support for the child with diabetes is imperative. The impact of hospitalization on a child is well documented. When Wilson and colleagues[9] encouraged hospitalized children to tell their stories, the investigators learned that loneliness and feeling scared were common themes. Rennick and Rashotte[10] found that children may not recall clear details of their PICU experience, but their perceptions are distorted by their limited or immature cognitive abilities. This leads to anxiety, which may persist well beyond the hospitalization.

The type of support PICU nurses should provide is best determined by the child's chronologic and developmental age. The very young child needs to feel safe and comforted, whereas the older child needs to have their autonomy and independence nurtured.[11] Even preschool children can begin to participate in self-care. Simply pushing the button on a BG meter or selecting the injection site and swabbing the site with alcohol can build early skills. It is important to recognize, however, that the young child will not want to perform these tasks every time.[12] For the older school-aged child and teen, learning self-care skills is imperative. During their stay in the PICU, they can become familiar with the necessary skills, but more extensive training and support is needed after discharge.

The often forgotten family member is the sibling. There is no doubt that siblings are affected by the diagnosis of diabetes.[13] Jackson and colleagues[14] suggested that "sibling perceptions of diabetes and parental distress are important predictors of sibling adjustment" (p. 308). There seems to be important links between the coping of all family members. Supporting the siblings might include visits to the PICU[15] or using technology (such as Skype) to connect the family.

COMPREHENSIVE DIABETES SELF-MANAGEMENT EDUCATION

Although survival skills and knowledge can help families through the initial days and weeks of managing diabetes, more extensive or comprehensive self-management education is needed to live successfully with diabetes. The National Standards for Diabetes Self-Management Education serve as a guide for the nurse or diabetes educator.[16] In addition, the American Association of Diabetes Educators (AADE) has developed guidelines and collected evidence to support 7 self-care behaviors specific to diabetes education.

A diabetes curriculum built on these 7 behaviors should address aspects of monitoring, medications, nutrition, activity, risk control, problem solving, and coping.[17] Evidence suggests that educating children and adolescents with diabetes may have "a modestly beneficial effect on glycemic control and a stronger effect on psychosocial outcomes."[18(p55)] Several published curricula are available, but the unique educational needs of children with diabetes must also be considered. Parents and other caregivers must be involved and the education must honor the developmental level of the child. In addition, ongoing diabetes self-management education must be provided as the child matures and is able to take on more self-care behaviors. Transitioning from parental care to self-care is yet another difference in a pediatric diabetes curriculum.[11,19]

Critical care nurses should encourage families to continue their education in the management of diabetes beyond the hospital care. There are many new strategies to help children and families learn about diabetes. Sullivan-Bolyai and colleagues[20] described a novel approach using simulation to help parents learn to manage acute situations in diabetes care. Computer games, such as Power Defense, are in development to help children react to diabetes scenarios in a format they prefer.[21] Diabetes summer camps afford a unique learning and support environment for children and teens with diabetes.

Hospitalization is not the opportune time to provide anything but survival information, and there is controversy about how much should even be addressed in the hospital or critical care unit.

HOW MUCH DIABETES SELF-MANAGEMENT EDUCATION SHOULD OCCUR IN THE HOSPITAL?

Siminerio and colleagues[22] demonstrated that comprehensive diabetes education can be provided effectively in the outpatient setting. Several years later, in a Cochrane Library review, the few available studies confirmed these findings.[23] In Beal and colleagues,[24] Gray advocated for a brief hospital stay at diagnosis to provide parents with support immediately around the diagnosis, whereas Doyle contended that outpatient education in a more natural setting is preferred for the child who is not critically ill. For the critical care nurse, it seems prudent to provide the basic survival education while assuring adequate follow-up and continued comprehensive training in the outpatient center. For Jack, the child described at the beginning of this article, basic survival skill training should be planned. Attention to the emotional needs of the child, his sibling, his parents, and his grandparents should be offered. Often a child life-program specialist or clinical nurse specialist can also support the critical care nurse in providing additional emotional support to the family.

SUPPORTING DIABETES EDUCATION: THE CRITICAL CARE NURSE'S ROLE

The critically ill child and family depend on the PICU nurse to monitor and evaluate physiologic changes and to act and react confidently to those changes. Critical care competencies focus on these skills. For the child with diabetes, additional competencies in the critical care nurse should include attention to building self-care skills when the time is right.

Competencies for managing diabetes include knowledge of nutrition, an understanding of BG excursions, technical skills in the use of meters, insulin pens, and insulin pumps, and patient education and coaching skills. Critical care nurses should also have a strong background in the management of hyperglycemia with insulin.[25] Refresher courses and skill updates may be required if the PICU does not admit many children with diabetes.[26]

Children who are diagnosed and immediately admitted to a PICU need the skills and knowledge of competent nursing staff. Parents also need to know that diabetes is a disease that is manageable and need nursing staff who skillfully return their child to a new state of normal. The PICU nurse is often the one to prepare the family for their first day at home with diabetes. Parents want to know what to feed their child, when to give insulin, what symptoms to pay attention to, and what to do next. The PICU nurse is in the position to provide clear instructions and ensure that the instructions are understood. For the child who is admitted to the PICU or hospital repeatedly, the story is different.

EDUCATING AND SUPPORTING THE CHILD WITH REPEATED ADMISSIONS

In 1 study, 46% of families responded that their child had been rehospitalized at some point after diagnosis of diabetes[27] although overall rates of hospitalization for children with diabetes have remained stable for more than a decade.[28] Several investigators have explored the question of why children are readmitted. Estrada and colleagues[27] viewed readmission as a failure of the outpatient management system for some children. Other investigators have attributed repeat hospitalizations to underlying psychiatric or emotional issues in the child or family.[29,30]

For instance, intentional insulin omission often results in rehospitalization and admission to the PICU. Adolescent girls, in particular, may withhold insulin as a way to lose weight.[31] The practice is often associated with depression and underlying family dysfunction. For the critical care nurse, careful assessment often uncovers the teen's unhealthy weight perception and lack of knowledge about risks in omitting insulin.[32]

In many cases, the hospitalized adolescent is well versed in diabetes skills and knowledge. Typically, the adolescent has stopped taking insulin and stopped monitoring care. Parents may not be engaged or supportive. As in the case of Janequa and her insulin pump at the beginning of this article, there may be a variety of resources available to the child, but they are not being used appropriately. Traditional diabetes self-management education may not be the answer. Coping skills and problem solving should be emphasized. The child may be dealing with peer pressure, hovering parents, or diabetes burnout, a common condition from the unrelenting demands of diabetes self-care.[33] After stabilizing the child hemodynamically, assessing carefully, and educating where needed, the critical care nurse's best approach is to enlist the help of mental health colleagues in approaching the teen's ineffective coping.

SUMMARY

Children with diabetes and their families present a unique challenge for the critical care nurse. Diabetes requires daily decision making about food, medication, activity, and BG levels. For the newly diagnosed child in the PICU, the primary concern is attending to the physical and physiologic needs. Ultimately, the family needs survival skills and knowledge to leave the hospital safely and confidently.

For the newly diagnosed child, the critical care nurse's role is to address safety, simple pathophysiology, skills, school, and support with children and families. Engaging the child and family in self-care skills helps with their coping and adapting. Including siblings in the child's care can also support emotional healing.

For the child or teen frequently readmitted to the PICU, the critical care nurse's priorities are to stabilize, assess, educate, and support the efforts of mental health colleagues in managing the underlying emotional issues. This article offered suggestions for the critical care nurse to begin helping these children and families acquire diabetes self-management skills, even in the PICU.

REFERENCES

1. Nettles AT. Patient education in the hospital. Diabetes Spectrum 2005;18:44–8.
2. White RO, Wolff K, Cavanaugh KL, et al. Addressing health literacy and numeracy to improve diabetes education and care. Diabetes Spectrum 2010; 23:238–43.
3. Osborn CY, Cavanaugh K, Kripalani S. Strategies to address low health literacy and numeracy in diabetes. Clin Diabetes 2010;28:171–5.
4. Van Scoyoc EE, DeWalt DA. Interventions to improve diabetes outcomes for people with low literacy and numeracy: a systematic literature review. Diabetes Spectrum 2010;23:228–37.
5. Lowes L, Gregory J, Line P. Newly diagnosed childhood diabetes: a psychosocial transition for parents? J Adv Nurs 2005;50:253–61.
6. Aldridge MD. Decreasing parental stress in the pediatric intensive care unit: one unit's experience. Crit Care Nurse 2005;25:40–50.
7. Marshall M, Carter B, Rose K, et al. Living with type 1 diabetes: perceptions of children and their parents. J Clin Nurs 2009;18:1703–10.
8. Whittemore R, Jaser S, Chao A, et al. Psychological experience of parents of children with type 1 diabetes: a systematic mixed-studies review. Diabetes Educ 2012;38:562–79.
9. Wilson ME, Megel ME, Enenbach L, et al. The voices of children: stories about hospitalization. J Pediatr Health Care 2010;24:95–102.
10. Rennick JE, Rashotte J. Psychological outcomes in children following pediatric intensive care unit hospitalization: a systematic review of the research. J Child Health Care 2009;13:128–49.

11. Schreiner B. Children with diabetes. In: Childs B, Cypress M, Spollett G, editors. Complete nurse's guide to diabetes care. 2nd edition. Alexandria (VA): American Diabetes Association; 2009. p. 340–66.
12. Halvorson M, Yasuda P, Carpenter S, et al. Unique challenges for pediatric patients with diabetes. Diabetes Spectrum 2005;18:167–73.
13. Hollidge C. Psychological adjustment of siblings to a child with diabetes. Health Soc Work 2001;26:15–25.
14. Jackson C, Richer J, Edge JA. Sibling psychological adjustment to type 1 diabetes mellitus. Pediatr Diabetes 2008;9:308–11.
15. Frazier A, Frazier H, Warren NA. A discussion of family-centered care within the pediatric intensive care unit. Crit Care Nurs Q 2010;33:82–6.
16. Haas L, Maryniuk M, Beck J, et al. National standards for diabetes self-management education and support. Diabetes Educ 2012;38:619–29.
17. American Association of Diabetes Educators (AADE). AADE guidelines for the practice of diabetes self-management education and training. Chicago(IL): AADE; 2011. Available at: http://www.diabeteseducator.org/export/sites/aade/_resources/pdf/general/PracticeGuidelines2011.pdf. Accessed September 1, 2012.
18. Swift PG. Diabetes education in children and adolescents. Pediatr Diabetes 2009;10:51–7.
19. Smaldone A, Lawlor M. Pediatric diabetes education: a family affair. In: Weinger K, Carver C, editors. Educating your patient with diabetes. New York: Humana Press; 2009. p. 251–71.
20. Sullivan-Bolyai S, Bova C, Lee M, et al. Parent education through simulation–diabetes. Diabetes Educ 2012;38:50–7.
21. Bassilious E, DeChamplain A, McCabe I, et al. Power defense: a video game for improving diabetes numeracy. In: CHI'12, Austin (TX): 2012. Available at: http://shared.uoit.ca/shared/faculty/fbit/documents/Student%20Achievements/Student%20Paper.pdf. Accessed September 1, 2012.
22. Siminerio L, Charron-Prochownik D, Banion C, et al. Comparing outpatient to inpatient diabetes education for newly diagnosed pediatric patients: a comprehensive measurement approach. Diabetes Educ 1999;25:895–906.
23. Clar C, Waugh N, Thomas S. Routine hospital admission versus out-patient or home care in children at diagnosis of type 1 diabetes mellitus. Cochrane Database Syst Rev 2007;(2):CD004099.
24. Beal J, Grey M, Doyle E. Should children with type 1 diabetes be hospitalized at diagnosis? MCN Am J Matern Child Nurs 2011;36:214–5.
25. Lange Zamudio V. Successful management of in-hospital hyperglycemia: the pivotal role of nurses in facilitating effective insulin use. Medsurg Nurs 2010; 119:323–8.
26. Manchester CS. Diabetes education in the hospital: establishing professional competency. Diabetes Spectrum 2008;21:268–71.
27. Estrada CL, Danielson KK, Drum ML, et al. Hospitalization subsequent to diagnosis in young patients with diabetes in Chicago, Illinois. Pediatrics 2009;124:926–34.
28. Lee JM, Okumura MJ, Freed GL, et al. Trends in hospitalizations for diabetes among children and young adults: United States, 1993–2004. Diabetes Care 2007;30:3035–9.
29. Garrison MM, Katon WJ, Richardson LP. The impact of psychiatric comorbidities on readmissions for diabetes in youth. Diabetes Care 2005;28:2150–4.
30. Lewin AB, Heidgerken AD, Geffken GR, et al. The relation between family factors and metabolic control: the role of diabetes adherence. J Pediatr Psychol 2006;31:174–83.

31. Ruth-Sahd LA, Schneider M, Haagen B. Diabulimia: what it is and how to recognize it in critical care. Dimens Crit Care Nurs 2009;28:147–53.
32. Howe CJ, Jawad AF, Kely SD, et al. Weight-related concerns and behaviors in children and adolescents with type I diabetes. J Am Psychiatr Nurses Assoc 2008;13:376–85.
33. Polonsky WH. Diabetes burnout. Alexandria (VA): American Diabetes Association; 1999.

Management of the Hospitalized Diabetes Patient with an Insulin Pump

Deborah McCrea, RN, MSN, CNS, CEN, CFRN, EMT-P

KEYWORDS

- Insulin pump • Continuous subcutaneous insulin infusion • Basal rate • Bolus rate
- Insulin to carbohydrate ratio • Correction factor/sensitivity factor

KEY POINTS

- More than 375,000 Americans with diabetes use an insulin pump.
- Many insulin-pump patients choose to wear the pump while hospitalized.
- The nurse needs to be familiar with insulin-pump therapy in the event that a patient is hospitalized wearing an insulin pump.

INTRODUCTION

Over the last 30 years, impressive improvements in technology have enhanced diabetes management for those who take insulin daily. Until the late 1970s, patients had few insulin types and brands from which to choose and only one way by which to deliver insulin (syringe). The first blood-glucose test strip was introduced in 1965, and years later the first glucose meter was introduced in 1971. It was not until home glucose monitoring was available that patients were able to intensify insulin therapy with the use of multiple daily injections (via syringe or insulin pen) or insulin pump. The first insulin pump was introduced onto the market in 1978.[1] It was very large (about the size of a brick) compared with today's small insulin pumps (about the size of a pager or cell phone). Patients can now deliver insulin more accurately and discreetly.

Types of insulin have improved. The first rapid-acting insulin analogue, lispro (Humalog), was introduced in 1996. Since then, 2 other rapid-acting insulin analogues and 2 basal insulin analogues have been introduced. Home glucose monitoring has improved over the years. Meters are now more accurate, take only a few seconds

Disclosure: The author currently works for Medtronic Diabetes, Inc. on a contract basis only, teaching insulin pump and glucose sensor customers how to use their new medical equipment.
Department of Emergency Medical Services, Houston Community College, 555 Community College Drive, Suite 117, Houston, TX 77013, USA
E-mail address: deborah.mccrea@hccs.edu

to produce a result, and require a very small sample size. Some meters are even able to check β-hydroxybutyrate (blood ketones). The newest technology comprises continuous interstitial-fluid glucose-monitoring devices that are valuable for their glucose trending information.

The number of patients using the insulin pump has dramatically increased since its introduction onto the United States market. The Food and Drug Administration estimated that in 2007 there were more than 375,000 people with diabetes who wear insulin pumps.[1,2] Graff and colleagues[3] conducted a survey of people who treat diabetes and also have diabetes, and found that 96% of diabetes specialists including physicians, nurse practitioners, physician assistants, and certified diabetes educators who have type 1 diabetes practiced intensive insulin management for their own diabetes. Of those practicing intensive management, more than half chose to wear an insulin pump.

Many who wear an insulin pump continue to use this technology even in the hospital setting; therefore, it is important for the nurse to understand the insulin pump. This article discusses the benefits of intensive insulin therapy, how the insulin pump works, initial insulin-pump dosing, candidate selection, advantages and disadvantages of using an insulin pump, nursing care of the hospitalized patient wearing an insulin pump, troubleshooting the insulin pump, and development of hospital protocols for caring for the patient wearing an insulin pump.

BENEFITS OF INTENSIVE INSULIN MANAGEMENT

Before the late 1970s, the relationship between poor glucose control and long-term diabetes complications was not well understood. The Diabetes Control and Complications Trial (DCCT), launched in 1982, was a 9-year landmark study involving 1441 patients with type 1 diabetes.[4,5] Trial participants who practiced intensive insulin management (using multiple daily insulin injections or the insulin pump) achieved lower levels of hemoglobin A1c and had 76% less diabetic retinopathy, 56% less diabetic nephropathy, and 60% less neuropathy compared with patients using nonintensive therapy. The Epidemiology of Diabetes Interventions and Complications (EDIC) was a follow-up study of the outcomes of the trial participants of the DCCT study,[5,6] which included 96% of the DCCT participants (N = 1357). The study looked at whether intensive insulin therapy over a long period of time reduced cardiovascular, advanced retinopathic, and nephropathic complications. The results of the EDIC trial showed that diabetes complications were significantly reduced in those DCCT trial participants who practice intensive insulin therapy. **Table 1** shows the reduction in risk for microvascular complications with intensive insulin therapy in comparison with conventional therapy during the DCCT and EDIC Trials.

DESCRIPTION OF THE INSULIN PUMP

An insulin pump is a small battery-operated external device that delivers insulin subcutaneously. The insulin pump uses rapid-acting insulin such as aspart (Novolog), lispro (Humalog), or glulisine (Apidra), or short-acting insulin (Regular). The rapid-acting insulin analogues are used in the insulin pump more commonly because the onset is approximately 15 minutes, compared with an onset of Regular insulin at 30 minutes to 1 hour. The insulin pump delivers a continuous subcutaneous infusion via a subcutaneous cannula that is changed every 3 days.[1,7] Various brands of insulin pumps are available on the United States market. Pumps can either be tubeless whereby the pump is activated via a remote device, or be attached directly to the patient via tubing. There are varieties of pump sizes, pump colors, infusion sets, cannula materials

Table 1
Reduction in risk for microvascular complications with intensive therapy, compared with conventional therapy, during the DCCT and EDIC trials

Complication	DCCT[a]	EDIC[b]
Retinopathy: 3-step change	63%	72%
Retinopathy: proliferative	47%	76%
Retinopathy: macular edema	26%	77%
Retinopathy: laser therapy	51%	77%
Nephropathy: microalbuminuria	39%	53%
Nephropathy: clinical albuminuria	54%	82%
Neuropathy	60%	

[a] $P<.001$ for all reductions, except for macular edema during DCCT, which was not significant.
[b] EDIC assessment of neuropathy was different from DCCT assessment, precluding comparison of DCCT and EDIC results.

(Teflon or steel), cannula sizes, adhesives, and various "bells and whistles" that the patient can choose, just as when purchasing their laptop or smart phone. **Table 2** lists the brands of insulin pump available on the United States market.[8,9] All of the pump manufactures have customer service departments that are open 24 hours daily to help troubleshoot the insulin pump and a Web site to view the features of the pump. Many have user guides that are available for download.

MODES OF OPERATION OF THE INSULIN PUMP

Insulin pumps have 2 main modes of operation to deliver insulin to the patient, known as the basal rate and the bolus dose.[10] The basal rate is a constant, continuous flow of

Table 2
Manufacturers of insulin pumps in the United States, 2012

Manufacturer	Pump Model	Web Site, Tel.
Roche	Accu-Chek Spirit	www.accu-chekinsulinpumps.com 1-800-688-4578
Animas–Johnson & Johnson	One Touch Ping	www.animas.com 1-877-937-7867
Sooil	Dana Diabecare IIS	www.sooilusa.com 1-866-747-6645
Medtronic MiniMed	Paradigm Real Time Revel	www.medtronicdiabetes.com 1-888-350-3199
Insulet Corporation	OmniPod Insulin Management System	www.myomnipod.com 1-800-591-3455
Nipro Diabetes Systems	Amigo	www.niprodiabetes.com 1-888-651-7867
Tandem Diabetes Care	Tandem	www.tandemdiabetes.com 1-877-801-6901

Data from Diabetes Health Journal Product Reference Guide. 2012. Available at: http://www.diabeteshealth.com/media/pdfs/PRG0112/Insulin%20Pumps%20Chart.pdf. Accessed August 24, 2012; and Diabetes Forecast Journal Consumer Guide Charts. 2012. Available at: http://forecast.diabetes.org/files/images/v65n01_Insulin_Pumps.pdf. Accessed August 24, 2012.

insulin that mimics the normal basal delivery of insulin from the patient's pancreas that occurred before being diagnosed with diabetes. Before pump therapy, patients use medium-term or longer-acting insulin for their basal needs. Insulin such as NPH (Neutral Protamine Hagedorn), glargine (Lantus), and detemir (Levemir) are examples of basal insulin.

Basal insulin, the insulin needed to metabolize the glucose secreted by the liver, is infused by the insulin pump continuously to maintain normoglycemia between meals and during sleep. The insulin pump can be programmed to deliver a variety of basal rates to meet the needs of the patient. Increased basal rates are needed for various factors including dawn phenomenon, stress, premenstrual times, certain medications causing hyperglycemia, and especially glucocorticoids. Dawn phenomenon is caused by the increases in growth hormone, cortisol, and epinephrine during the second half of the sleep cycle. Most adults, starting at puberty, will need an increase in the basal rate during the second half of their sleep cycle until mid-morning and then a reduction in basal rate close to noontime, followed by a gradual increase in the afternoon.[10] Once the basal rates have been set correctly, in theory no additional insulin is needed for a fasting individual.[11]

A bolus rate is used to maintain blood-glucose levels after meals or snacks or to correct high levels during times of illness, additional stress, or miscalculation of previous dosages that have caused high blood glucose.[11]

INITIAL DOSAGE CALCULATION FOR BASAL AND BOLUS RATES

The most common approach to calculating the initial total insulin-pump dose is to add the prepump total daily dose of all insulin units injected daily and then reduce that number by 25%. Of the total pump dose, approximately 50% will be the total basal dose and approximately 50% will be the total bolus dose. The total basal dose is then divided by 24 to obtain a starting basal rate per hour. The total bolus dose is divided between the 3 meals or, alternatively, the insulin to carbohydrate ratio (ICR) is calculated. The most common formula used to calculate the initial ICR is the 500 Rule, calculated by dividing the prepump total insulin dose by 500 to obtain the initial ICR. For example, if a patient was using a total of 60 units of insulin per day before starting on the insulin pump, the starting ICR would be 1 unit per 8 g of carbohydrate $(500 \div 60 = 8.3)$.[10–13]

If the blood glucose is higher than the target, the sensitivity factor (also known as the correction factor) is used to treat hyperglycemia. There are several mathematical formulas by which to calculate an initial sensitivity factor, used according to prescriber preference. For example, if the prescriber chooses the 1700 Rule for the initial sensitivity factor and the patient was using 60 units of insulin before starting on the insulin pump, the initial sensitivity factor would be 28 $(1700 \div 60 = 28.33)$.[10–13]

The ICR and the sensitivity factor is programmed into the insulin pump. The patient counts grams of carbohydrate and checks the blood-glucose levels before eating. The patient inputs the data into the insulin pump, and the insulin pump calculates the correct dose.[10–13] **Box 1** lists the steps required to calculate the starting dosages for insulin pumps.

Another variable programmed into the pump is the active insulin time, which is the duration of a bolus. The duration varies depending on the type of insulin used in the pump. Most patients select 4 to 6 hours. The pump keeps track of the amount of insulin bloused within the programmed active insulin time. If the patient wants to take a bolus to correct hyperglycemia, the insulin pump will reduce the dose or even recommend no bolus if the patient has recently bolused. This feature reduces

---

Box 1

Steps to calculate starting dosages for insulin pumps

1. Calculate the prepump total daily dose (TDD) by adding the number of units of insulin injected per day before starting on the insulin pump

2. Calculate the pump TDD by reducing the prepump TDD by 25%

3. Calculate the total basal dose by dividing the pump TDD in half. Divide the total basal dose by 24 to obtain the hourly basal rate.

4. Calculate the total bolus dose by dividing the pump TDD in half. Divide the total bolus dose by 3 to obtain the dose per meal, or calculate the insulin to carbohydrate ratio (ICR) using the 500 Rule.

5. To calculate the initial ICR, divide the prepump TDD by 500

6. To calculate the initial sensitivity factor (SF), divide the prepump TDD by 1700

For example:

- Prepump TDD: 60 units/d

- Pump TDD (with 25% reduction) = 45 units/d

- Basal rate: $45 \div 2 = 22.5$ units/d (0.93 units/h)

- Bolus Rate: $45 \div 2 = 22.5$; then $\div$ by 3 meals = 7.5 units/meal

- ICR: $500 \div 60 = 8.3$ (so 1 unit is given)

- CF: $1700 \div 60 = 28$ (so 1 unit will reduce blood glucose by 28 mg/dL)

Data from Refs.[10–13]

---

the risk of "stacking" insulin boluses, which could cause hypoglycemia. All 3 rapid-acting insulin analogues described previously have similar action curves, with an onset occurring in 5 to 15 minutes, a peak in 45 to 90 minutes, and an overall duration of about 3 to 4 hours.[10–13]

PATIENT SELECTION

Insulin pumps do require considerable dedication on the part of both patients and caregivers. Characteristics of a successful insulin-pump patient include being motivated to manage diabetes; having realistic expectations of pump therapy; demonstrating the ability to test blood glucose, count carbohydrate, and solve problems; being willing to learn; welcoming a challenge; having family support; being able to afford pump therapy; and being capable of comprehending the training and technical aspects of the pump.[13–16] Insulin-pump patients must be able to troubleshoot pump problems after initiation. Infrequently pumps can malfunction and require replacement, which forces a patient to rapidly resume insulin injections pending arrival of a new pump. Patients can experience catheter occlusions that interrupt the flow of insulin. For this reason, patients must be especially cognizant of their glucose levels and be prepared to change their insulin infusion set to address recurrent unexplained hyperglycemia. Patients must be good troubleshooters. Because insulin pumps can be labor intensive and technically challenging, careful patient selection is one of the most important elements in successful pump therapy.[7,10–16] **Box 2** lists medical indications for the insulin pump.

Box 2
Medical indications for an insulin pump

- Patient's desire to use the insulin pump to improve glycemic control
- Inadequate glycemic control despite multiple daily injections
- Frequent hypoglycemia and hyperglycemia, and diabetic ketoacidosis
- Unawareness of hypoglycemia
- Pregnancy
- Extreme insulin sensitivity, especially in babies and toddlers
- Dawn phenomenon
- Prepregnancy planning and conception
- Long-term microvascular and macrovascular diabetes complications
- Gastroparesis: pumps can slow down bolus dose to better match a slow gut motility

ADVANTAGES OF INSULIN-PUMP THERAPY

There are many advantages of using an insulin pump.[10–13,15] The major benefit is the customization of the basal and bolus doses to match the needs of the patient. Many variables can alter blood glucose such as food intake, exercise, weight, illness, hormonal fluctuation, circadian rhythms, growth spurts, pregnancy, menses, stress, illness, surgery, and certain medications, among many others. The insulin pump can be reprogrammed quickly to meet the changing requirements of the patient. It can deliver doses as small as 0.025 units per hour and it delivers more accurately than other insulin-delivery devices such as syringes, which helps reduce the risk of hypoglycemia. Patients who wear the insulin pump have more flexibility in the timing and amount of food consumed and in their lifestyle. The basal rate of the pump can be programmed to increase or decrease throughout the day and night to match the patient's basal requirements. For children, the pump can easily be programmed to change during growth cycles or changing hormones during puberty. The insulin pump can be used by athletes or exercisers to decrease insulin delivery either during or after exercise. The bolus doses can be delivered over a long period of time to allow for slowly digested foods such as high-fat meals. The insulin pump can be programmed to match the insulin needs for varied work schedules, traveling, exercise, stress, menses, illness, pregnancy, surgery, and so forth. The pump also calculates the insulin dose correctly, reducing mathematical errors in calculating premeal insulin doses. Insulin-pump patients have also been shown to gain less weight than those on multiple daily injections.[10–16] **Table 3** lists the advantages and disadvantages of insulin-pump therapy.

DISADVANTAGES OF INSULIN-PUMP THERAPY

Insulin-pump therapy has some disadvantages.[10–16] Because the pump only uses rapid-acting or short-acting insulin, if insulin delivery is disrupted then hyperglycemia and diabetic ketoacidosis may occur quickly. It is imperative that the insulin-pump patient knows the protocols for hyperglycemia and prevention of diabetic ketoacidosis, and how to troubleshoot and solve problems quickly. The insulin pump is a mechanical device that needs to be programmed, and some patients have difficulty learning how to program the pump as well as the rules that accompany the wearing of

Table 3	
Advantages and disadvantages of insulin-pump therapy	
Advantages	**Disadvantages**
Improves glycemic control	Potential for rapid onset of hyperglycemia
Offers precise dosage delivery	and diabetic ketoacidosis if insulin delivery
Can be programmed to increase or decrease	is interrupted
to follow circadian rhythms	Learning how to use the insulin pump
Allows for changes needed during growth or	Learning how to count grams of
changes	carbohydrate
Ideal for athletics/exercise to decrease insulin	Learn how to troubleshoot insulin-pump
delivery either during event or afterward	problems
Varied and prolonged bolusing for high-fat	Site infection (not common)
meals	Cost
Flexibility for varied work schedules, exercise	
regimens, flexible meal schedule	
Helpful for multiple time-zone travel	
Improves psychological well-being and	
quality of life	
Assists with better pre-/postmeal blood sugar	
levels	
Convenience of delivery of insulin	
Avoids 3–4 injections/d	
No math, owing to bolus calculators	
Weight control by avoiding extra snacks	

the pump. Patients must learn how to count grams of carbohydrate so that they receive the correct bolus dose. Infusion-site infections of the skin, although uncommon, can occur. Some patients can develop scar tissue from the insulin over time that can cause insulin-absorption problems and no-delivery alarms. Cost can be a barrier if the patient does not have adequate insurance coverage or financial resources to afford insulin-pump therapy.

USE OF THE INSULIN PUMP IN HOSPITALIZED PATIENTS

The American Academy of Clinical Endocrinology and the American Diabetes Association updated a consensus statement on inpatient glycemic management.[17] This consensus paper addresses the use of an insulin pump in hospitalized patients. Unfortunately most hospitals, because of a lack of staff understanding of pump therapy, and the lack of hospital policy and procedures, mandatorily force the insulin-pump patient to revert back to injections. Hospital policy and procedures outlining care of the hospitalized patient wearing an insulin pump should therefore be developed and implemented. Several hospitals around the country have developed and implemented policy and procedures for the care of the hospitalized insulin-pump patient.[18–25] These programs have similar frameworks comprising responsibilities of patients, medical staff, and prescribers, care of the hospitalized patient with an insulin pump, and troubleshooting the insulin pump (**Table 4**).

Patient Responsibility

The patient must be responsible for managing the insulin pump during hospitalization. Patient responsibilities include providing information to the health care team for the current pump settings, bringing in all necessary pump supplies, willingness to use the hospital's insulin, to use the hospital blood-glucose meter, to change the infusion

Table 4
Patient responsibilities, nursing responsibilities, and prescriber responsibilities

Patient Responsibilities	Nursing Responsibilities	Prescriber Responsibilities
Be able to physically operate the insulin pump	Perform an initial and ongoing assessment of the patient for the appropriateness of using the insulin pump	Perform an initial and ongoing assessment of the patient for the appropriateness of using the insulin pump
Be able to count carbohydrate, bolus correctly, and change the infusion set when needed	Perform blood-glucose monitoring	Write clear orders for the insulin type, all insulin pump settings, when to check blood glucose, and when to notify the prescriber for issues such as hypoglycemia, hyperglycemia, and situations that require changes in the insulin orders
Be willing to follow the hyperglycemia protocol	Document all blood-glucose results, boluses, and basal rates	
Have all necessary insulin-pump supplies at the hospital	Ensure the patient changes the infusion set every 72 h or more often if needed	
Be willing to have blood glucose checked as often as needed to achieve good glycemic control	Notify the prescriber if the insulin pump needs to be discontinued and an alternative insulin regimen needs to be prescribed	
Be willing to program the insulin pump according to the prescriber's orders		

set every 72 hours or more often if needed, and to refrain from changing any pump settings without an order from the prescriber.

Medical Staff Responsibility

The nurse needs to perform an initial and ongoing assessment of the patient, assessing for the appropriateness an insulin pump for the patient. If the nurse identifies a contraindication to the use of an insulin pump, the nurse will notify the authorized prescriber, obtain an alternative insulin order, and administer the prescribed regimen before using the insulin pump. The nurse needs to document all bolus and basal doses, perform blood glucose tests, and assess the infusion set and ensure it is changed at a minimum of every 72 hours. The prescriber must assess the appropriateness of the patient as regards wearing an insulin pump in hospital. If the patient is appropriate, clear orders must be written regarding insulin type, all insulin-pump settings, when blood glucose is to be checked, and when the prescriber should be notified about issues such as hypoglycemia, hyperglycemia, and situations that require changes in the insulin orders.

Troubleshooting Insulin-Pump Problems

One of the most common problems in all insulin users no matter how the insulin is injected (via syringe, pen, or insulin pump), is hyperglycemia. Many variables can cause hyperglycemia, as discussed earlier. The difference in troubleshooting hyperglycemia between in insulin-pump patients and those who use a syringe or pen is the infusion set. The insulin-pump infusion set can become bent, clogged, or dislodged, or may be impeded by scar tissue. All pump patients and their families should know the "hyperglycemia protocol."[10,12,13,15,16] When patients encounter an elevated blood-glucose level of more than 250 mg/dL, they should immediately take a correction bolus via the insulin pump and then recheck their blood glucose in 1 hour to make sure it is decreasing. If the blood glucose is decreasing, no further action is necessary. If the blood glucose in 1 hour is the same or higher than the previous blood glucose, patients should then take another correction dose via a syringe-based or pen-based system, not via the insulin pump. The blood glucose needs to be rechecked then in 1 hour. If the blood glucose is decreasing after 1 hour, patients should change the infusion set using new insulin. If this blood-glucose level is the same or higher the insulin could be deactivated, and patients may become dehydrated or ill. Patients should then administer an injection with new insulin, and immediately call their health care provider or go to the emergency room.

Hyperglycemia protocol

1. If the blood-glucose level is above 250 mg/dL, take a correction bolus via insulin pump.
2. Recheck blood glucose in 1 hour.
3. If the repeat blood-glucose level is decreasing, no further action is necessary.
4. If the repeat blood-glucose level is the same or higher, immediately take a correction dose via insulin syringe or pen.
5. Recheck the blood glucose in 1 hour.
6. If the repeat blood-glucose level is decreasing, change the infusion set and reservoir using new insulin. Recheck the blood glucose in 2 hours to make sure the new infusion set is working properly.
7. If the repeat blood-glucose level is the same or higher, the insulin may be bad, or dehydration or illness may be present. Take another injection using new insulin and contact the health care provider immediately, or go to the nearest emergency room.

When to Disconnect the Insulin Pump

There are times when the hospitalized insulin-pump patient must not be allowed to wear the pump. The pump needs to be discontinued if the patient is going to receive radiation or magnetic resonance imaging (MRI).[23,24,26] The patient should wear the insulin pump to the procedure and disconnect immediately before it begins. The medical staff will secure the insulin pump away from the radiation or MRI. If the procedure lasts less than 60 minutes, no adjustments or orders are needed. If the insulin pump is to be disconnected for more than 60 minutes, the prescriber will need to write orders for blood-glucose monitoring and treatment of hyperglycemia via insulin syringe or pen. The insulin pump needs to be discontinued if the patient is severely dehydrated. The patient will not absorb subcutaneous insulin and therefore will require an insulin drip. The insulin pump can be resumed once the dehydration is corrected, but the insulin pump will need to be started before discontinuing an insulin drip because the half-life of intravenous insulin is very short. The insulin pump needs to be discontinued if the patient is suicidal, critically ill, has altered mental status, or is unable or unwilling to adhere to hospital policy regarding the use of insulin pumps in the hospital.[27]

Special Situations

The insulin pump is often continued throughout procedures, during labor and delivery, and during surgery. The prescriber needs to assess the patient's pump settings and take into account factors such as the duration of fasting and whether the current pump settings are appropriate for the upcoming event. Questions to consider regard whether the upcoming event will cause a stress-hormone response leading to hyperglycemia, whether prolonged fasting will lead to hypoglycemia, and whether the patient will be able to operate the insulin pump after the procedure. The insulin pump may need to be either programmed to run at a temporary basal rate or reprogrammed for the event. In some instances the pump may need to be temporarily disconnected, and subcutaneous insulin injections ordered. The patient should have a fresh infusion site, distant enough so as not to interfere with the procedure or surgery. For example, laboring women may need to find an alternative site other than their abdomen or gluteal area in case there has to be an emergency cesarean section.

Development of Hospital Policy

When developing hospital policy and procedures regarding the care of the hospitalized patient with an insulin pump, one must first identify the issues and then gather input from the stakeholders before developing policies. The development of computerized order sheets can be produced from the policies. It will also be necessary to develop an education plan for the nursing and provider staff so that all of the medical staff understand what is expected from them.

SUMMARY

Almost 400,000 patients wear an insulin pump in the United States. Because many of these patients wish to continue wearing their pump during hospitalization, hospitals need to understand insulin-pump therapy, and write policies and procedures to safely manage the hospitalized insulin-pump patient. Both medical staff and patients need to understand and comply with hospital policies and procedures.

REFERENCES

1. Federal Drug Administration. General Hospital and Personal Use Medical Devices Panel Meeting, March 5, 2010. Available at: http://www.fda.gov/downloads/AdvisoryCommittees/CommitteesMeetingMaterials/MedicalDevices/MedicalDevicesAdvisoryCommittee/GeneralHospitalandPersonalUseDevicesPanel/UCM202779.pdf. Accessed November 23, 2012.
2. Lee S. History of pump technology. Medscape nurses education. Available at: http://www.medscape.org/viewarticle/460365_2. Accessed August 24, 2012.
3. Graff MR, Rubin RR, Walker EA. How diabetes specialists treat their own diabetes: findings from a study of the AADE and ADA membership. Diabetes Educ 2000;26(3):460–7.
4. The Diabetes Control and Complications Trial Research Group. The effect of intensive therapy of diabetes on the development and progression of long-term complications in insulin-dependent diabetes mellitus. N Engl J Med 1993;329(14):977–86.
5. U.S. Department of Health and Human Services, National Diabetes Information Clearinghouse (NDIC). Available at: http://diabetes.niddk.nih.gov/dm/pubs/control/DCCT-EDIC_508.pdf. Accessed August 24, 2012.
6. Epidemiology of Diabetes Interventions and Complications (EDIC): design, implementation, and preliminary results of a long-term follow-up of th1e Diabetes Control and Complications Trial Cohort. Diabetes Care 1999;22(1):99–111.
7. Warshaw H. Rapid-acting insulin timing it just right. Available at: http://www.diabetesselfmanagement.com/articles/insulin/rapid_acting_insulin/all. Accessed August 24, 2012.
8. Diabetes health journal product reference guide. 2012. Available at: http://www.diabeteshealth.com/media/pdfs/PRG0112/Insulin%20Pumps%20Chart.pdf. Accessed August 24, 2012.
9. Diabetes forecast journal consumer guide charts. 2012. Available at: http://forecast.diabetes.org/files/images/v65n01_Insulin_Pumps.pdf. Accessed August 24, 2012.

10. Skylar JS. The insulin pump therapy book: insights from the experts. Los Angeles (CA): MiniMed Inc; 1995.
11. Davidson PC. The insulin pump therapy book: insights from the experts. Los Angeles (CA): MiniMed Inc; 1995.
12. Bode BW. Pumping protocols, a guide to insulin pump therapy initiation. Medtronic diabetes. Available at: http://professional.medtronicdiabetes.com. Accessed August 24, 2012.
13. Scheiner G. Insulin pump therapy: guidelines for successful outcomes. American Association of Diabetes Educators 2008 Consensus Summit. Chicago, September 18, 2008.
14. Beaser RS, Staff of Joslin Diabetes Center. Joslin's insulin deskbook, designing and initiation insulin treatment program. Boston: Joslin Diabetes Center; 2008. Accessed August 24, 2012.
15. Scheiner G. Think like a pancreas, a practical guide to managing diabetes with insulin. Cambridge (MA): Da Capo Press; 2004.
16. Jovanovic-Peterson L, Peterson CM. Planting the Pump. Diabetes Professional 1990;23–37.
17. Moghissi ES, Korytkowski MT, DiNardo M, et al. American Association of Clinical Endocrinologists and American Diabetes Association consensus statement on inpatient glycemic control. Diabetes Care 2009;32:1119–31.
18. Lee SW, Im R, Magbual R. Current perspectives on the use of continuous subcutaneous insulin infusion in the acute care setting and overview of therapy. Crit Care Nurs Q 2004;27:172–84.
19. Wesorick D, O'Malley C, Rushakoff R, et al. Management of diabetes and hyperglycemia in the hospital: a practical guide to subcutaneous insulin use in the non-critically ill, adult patient. Society of Hospital Medicine Web site. Available at: http://www.hospitalmedicine.org/ResourceRoomRedesign/html/04Best_Practices/03_Managing_Diabetes.cfm. Accessed August 24, 2012.
20. Cook B, Boyle ME, Cisar NS, et al. Use of continuous subcutaneous insulin infusion therapy in the hospital setting: proposed guidelines and outcome measures. Diabetes Educ 2005;31:849–57.
21. Bailon PW, Partlow BJ, Miller-Cage V, et al. Continuous subcutaneous insulin infusion (insulin pump) therapy can be safely used in the hospital in select patients. Endocr Pract 2009;15:24–9.
22. Noshes ML, DiNardo MM, Donahue AC, et al. Patient outcomes after implementation of a protocol for inpatient insulin pump therapy. Endocr Pract 2009;15:415–24.
23. JHH Glucose Management Committee. Insulin pumps in the hospital. Available at: http://www.hopkinsmedicine.org/endocrinology/diabetes/inpatient_diabetes_management_service/Insulin_Pumps_Hospital.pdf. Accessed August 24, 2012.
24. Joslin Diabetes Center. Joslin Clinic guidelines for inpatient management of surgical and ICU patients with diabetes (pre, peri and postoperative care). Available at: http://www.joslin.org/docs/Inpatient_Guideline_10-02-09.pdf. Accessed August 24, 2012.
25. Ran JJ, Holden RL. A practical guide to insulin pump management in adults in and around hospital. Available at: http://www.diabetes.ca/documents/for-professionals/CD-Autumn_2011–R.Houlden_.pdf. Accessed August 24, 2012.
26. Marks JB. Perioperative management of diabetes. Am Fam Physician 2003;67:93–100.
27. McCrea DL, McCrea CA. Emergency department care of the patient with an insulin pump. J Emerg Nurs 1991;17:220–4.

Critical Care Diabetes Education
Who, What, When, Where, and Why

Judy Keaveny, RN, MSN, CNS M-S, CDE

KEYWORDS

- Diabetes • Diabetes education • Diabetes medications • Insulin • Hyperglycemia
- Hypoglycemia • Insulin resistance

KEY POINTS

- Studies are confirming that adequate education decreases hospitalization rates for patients with diabetes and hyperglycemia initially and long term for acute and chronic complications, readmissions, and extended length of stay.
- Patients need to be identified early, by evaluating the glucose and hemoglobin A1C levels of patients with steroids, infection, sepsis, wounds, high blood pressure, or known diabetes.
- Critical care nurses need to be involved, starting basic education about what diabetes is; symptoms; causes and treatment; monitoring; insulin; injections; goals for glucose levels; prevention of infection; and the balance of food, diet, medication, and exercise.

INTRODUCTION

Hyperglycemia occurs in hospitalized patients both with and without diabetes, especially if they are treated with steroids. From 41% to 56% of patients without diabetes treated with steroids and 75% to 81% of patients with diabetes treated with steroids experience hyperglycemia.[1] With the increasing rate of diabetes in the population, which reached about 8.5% in 2011, and increasing obesity, it is essential that blood glucose levels are monitored and evaluated during and after their acute illness.[2] Insulin resistance and stress hormones are key components when stressors, surgery, trauma, infection, medical disease, and myocardial infarction occur.[3] Stress diabetes presents when triggers such as increased cortisol, catecholamines, glucagon, growth hormone, gluconeogenesis, and glycogenolysis increase blood glucose.[4] Many people have undiagnosed type 2 diabetes, making it difficult to determine whether hyperglycemia is a result of only stress hormones or whether the patient has diabetes.

Disclosure: The author has no relationship with a commercial company that has a direct financial interest in the subject matter or materials discussed in this article, or with a company making a competing product.
Department of General Internal Medicine, The University of Texas MD Anderson Cancer Center, 1515 Holcombe, Mail Code 0332, Houston, TX 77030, USA
E-mail address: jkeaveny@mdanderson.org

Crit Care Nurs Clin N Am 25 (2013) 123–130
http://dx.doi.org/10.1016/j.ccell.2012.11.006
0899-5885/13/$ – see front matter Published by Elsevier Inc.

Additional laboratory testing with hemoglobin A1C (HbA1C) may be helpful.[5] These hormones and insulin resistance are present during even minor surgery or events, but can often continue uncontrolled with major events.[6]

Initial education and understanding that they need regular follow-up are essential points to explain to patients, their families, and significant others. Understanding that diabetes is a family disease helps them make learning more meaningful. Patients also realize that they can be an example to their families, with some coaching. They realize that their children and grandchildren need to start making changes early in life. This discussion point can be a motivator for their learning and later changes in behavior.

Start a discussion with understanding basic survival skills, as used by diabetes educators for many years: type of diabetes, monitoring, glucose goals, insulin, medications, and prevention of acute complications. Understanding the balance of these takes time but is important before discharge.

More commonly called diabetes self-management education (DSME) by health care team members, assessment and education include addressing the educational, clinical, behavioral, and emotional needs of each individual patient in a supportive environment. The overall objectives of diabetes self-management are to support informed decision making, self-care behaviors, problem solving, healthy coping, and active collaboration with the health care team. The results are improved clinical outcomes, health status, and quality of life. An initial Web site for patients to find free initial information and order booklets is www.YourDiabetesInfo.org.[7,8]

Become a leader by developing your teaching skills with hyperglycemic patients, with or without diagnosed diabetes. Identify who, what, when, where, and why. The goals for each patient vary depending on the type of diabetes or the causes of hyperglycemia. A patient with diabetic ketoacidosis secondary to newly diagnosed type 1 diabetes, a type 2 diabetic with severe dehydration or nonketotic hyperosmolar state, and a patient with steroid-induced diabetes all have different goals and needs. Most patients get scared by all the talk. The more they understand what and why this has happened, the less fearful they become, making learning easier for them. There are sometimes even threats from family or staff such as "You don't want to lose your foot, do you?" This is not acceptable teaching, because instilling fear decreases the ability to learn. They are still feeling ill, and it happened so quickly? They may be saying, "Surely, I won't need insulin, will I?" This may be their biggest fear. A new patient with hyperglycemia should be taught with basic facts and a focus on what they can do to get better, how to stay that way, and the resources that are available.[9]

What do patients need to know before discharge? The American Association of Diabetes Educators (AADE) have researched and identified self-care behaviors to help coordinate the multifaceted and individualized education that is needed. These behaviors are called AADE7 Self-Care Behaviors. These 7 key behaviors include healthy eating, being active, monitoring, taking medication, problem solving, healthy coping, and reducing risks. Various teaching tools and handouts have been developed and include individualization within each area. There are patient handouts that can be printed from their Web site: www.diabeteseducator.org.

Where do you start? Most patients need monitoring of glucose levels, goals for their glucose levels, and what to do when the levels are high or low. Start medication and insulin administration as soon as possible, but they may not be ready at first.[9]

WHO SHOULD BE TARGETED?

Identify patients who are newly hyperglycemic or newly diagnosed with or without ketoacidosis, or those who are on steroids with glucose levels more than 140 mg/dL, new infections or sepsis, and those patients with known diabetes but with increased emergency center or admission glucose levels. Check whether a recent HbA1C has been done; if more than 6.4%, they need further evaluation for contributing factors. Teaching these factors can help prevent future reoccurrences. Infection is another factor that raises glucose levels, indicating possible type 2 diabetes and some insulin resistance if the glucose levels are more than 140 mg/dL. Recommendation for steroid-induced hyperglycemia is to be retested 30 days after finishing the steroids, to evaluate whether the patient has any continued glucose increases. If so, follow-up glucose tests are recommended, to confirm with 2 laboratory tests to determine whether diagnostic levels are reached for prediabetes or diabetes.[5] Understanding prediabetes diagnosis criteria also helps to identify patients earlier. Prediabetes criteria for diagnosis are if the fasting glucose is 100 mg/dL to 125 mg/dL or 2-hour postprandial glucose is 140 mg/dL to199 mg/dL, or HbA1C is 5.7% to 6.4%. Diabetes diagnostic criteria are when the fasting glucose is 126 mg/dL or higher, 2-hour postprandial is 200 mg/dL or higher, or HbA1C 6.5% or higher. Identifying prediabetes is a way to get education and treatment earlier and has been shown to slow the progression of diabetes to type 2 diabetes. In summary, identify patients with increased admission glucose levels, infection of any kind, sepsis, surgery, acute myocardial infarction or known heart disease, high cholesterol tests, hypertension, respiratory illness with steroid administration, or new wounds that are slow to heal. Check that glucose tests are done, and, if not, request HbA1C.[5]

In a 2010 study by Morrison,[10] from Columbia University School of Nursing, New York, of patients with postpancreatic resection for pancreatic cancer, critical care nurses were the first-line providers and assessed and managed acute complications in addition to educating patients about the long-term complications and management of these complications. Critical care nurses can be leaders as the first-line providers, and have an impact on patients' life-long control.

WHAT TO TEACH?

Start with simple explanations of what is happening with a patient's insulin, pancreas, and insulin resistance because of the body's uncontrolled hormone release, heredity factors, insulin meal scale, basal and bolus insulin doses, and dosage requirements. Basal (longer acting) insulin covers muscle needs. Bolus insulin doses covers food as it is digested, because the pancreas is slow to release enough. What does insulin resistance mean? Use familiar examples, to help patients understand. For example, glucose (from food that is broken down) is the fuel for the body, as gasoline is to a car. To go faster, the car needs more gasoline. As you have increased needs, you need more insulin to get the glucose to the muscles. Remember to let patients do some of the talking, to get familiar with their questions. They are usually concerned with their food. Be sure that they consult a dietitian before discharge. Let patients know when insulin doses change and why. Help them understand the normal levels for glucose, what their glucose numbers are, and their goals during their hospital stay. Their goals will be higher than normal glucose levels, and these goals may change later because of many factors. Help patients understand that HbA1C can be equated to an average glucose for 3 months. If they have a meter that displays averages, it helps patients to watch their numbers and relate them to a follow-up HbA1C. Nurses can start by learning basic diabetes education principles at the AADE Web site: www.diabeteseducator.org. Nurses do not need to be certified in diabetes to teach basic diabetes education, but they should keep current.[11]

A monitoring symposium was done in 2011 to address barriers to monitoring for people with diabetes and related conditions. Specific recommendations were developed by the participants, which included that people with diabetes benefit from instruction and guidance about self-monitoring and decision making that is based on monitored results and informed interactions with their providers. Collaboration within the diabetes care community is needed to ensure that monitoring is performed and used to its fullest advantage.[12]

Identifying barriers in diabetes self-management is another key element. Fear of hypoglycemia is expressed by many patients who use insulin. In 2007, Wild and colleagues[13] did a critical review of literature from 1985 to 2007 of English printed journals on fear of hypoglycemia in diabetes. Fear of hypoglycemia was found in 34 journals; a measurement scale was also identified, the Hypoglycemic Fear Survey. This scale addresses several factors that relate to whether an individual is likely to develop fear, such as whether there is a history of hypoglycemia, length of time since first insulin treatment, and a higher level of variability in blood glucose level. They concluded that there is evidence that fear of hypoglycemia may have a significant negative impact on diabetes management, metabolic control, and subsequent health outcomes. There is evidence that glucose awareness training and cognitive behavioral training can reduce levels of fear and improve disease management.[13]

WHEN: TIME, RESOURCES, AND OPPORTUNITY

A critical care unit often does not seem the best educational arena. Time and resources are limited, but opportunities can happen, such as every time a family comes to visit, or when you give an insulin injection or steroid medication, or possibly when an antibiotic is given. Are these teaching opportunities being explored? Relating treatment to what is happening to glucose or blood sugar helps patients to learn new terms. Answer questions about their intravenous (IV) glucose or insulin, and how it works. Help them recognize that they may have had symptoms for weeks or months, so discuss the typical symptoms.

Focus on 1 topic daily, or per shift if the patient can absorb it. Short stays in the critical care and surgery units are common, but communicate where patients are when they are transferred. Develop the care plan to help keep the communication on track for the best experience for the patient and family. Where is the patient in understanding the disease(s)? Frequent feedback of what has been learned so far is helpful. Patients have many new medical terms to learn. Are there booklets and videos available for the family to get them started, if the patient is not able? It is a family disease. Many free booklets can be ordered for your unit from the government Web site: http://diabetes.niddk.nih.gov/or private sources: www.healthyi.com/patient/diabetes. Pictures are helpful; most people are not sure where their pancreas is located.

Be sure your health care team knows what key principles your area will be focusing on. Having patients do their first self-injection eases many fears. Stock the smallest needles to allay their fears. Shorter needles may help them psychologically, too. Early hospital education has been shown to decrease length of stay.[14] Early referral to the diabetes educator is helpful, if available in your hospital. Have a resource list developed for areas in which patients need to continue their education, and attend a diabetes education program.

Learning new skills may the better starting point, such as the first injection of insulin, or doing a practice injection with saline, if on IV drip. People often have ideas, myths, misconceptions, and barriers about taking insulin. For example, they may say, "My mother died when she started insulin..." Find out what they know or think that they know, and start there. One of the most common questions that I receive is, "Do I have to be on insulin for the rest of my life?" If they have type 1 diabetes, the answer is "Yes," but explain why they need it, what ketoacidosis is, what could happen if they miss an injection, when to call the doctor, and how quickly they can develop ketoacidosis if left untreated. Getting them then to do their first injection usually helps. Can the family do the first injection for them? "Of course," I say. They need to have some say in what is happening. However, usually before discharge, they need to do a self-injection, unless they are very ill or debilitated. Explain this to them from the beginning, so that there are no surprises.

WHERE... CAN YOU MAKE A DIFFERENCE?

Many factors are involved in teaching and motivating behavior change, especially because major change is needed for many with diabetes. Educational levels of patients vary from illiterate, elementary level, or college, to beyond master's degrees. Cultural ideas about medicine, food, and lifestyle are crucial too. Start slowly and evaluate patients' comprehension of the basic concepts: glucose, insulin, and food that needs to be in balance. Repetition is needed, because average adults need to hear or do things 6 times to learn it. Recognize denial of having diabetes; statements like, "I refuse to let this sugar stay up", or "I don't want to have this, so I just won't." Listen to their comments to their families about what they are learning. Let them stay in control of what they think is most important to them. Food questions frequently come up, such as, "Can I still eat...?" There are near divorces over food! What people like and do not like is very personal. What are they willing to give up or not change? They usually voice these concerns. Some may have questions about travel, if their job requires it. Some may fear that, if started on insulin, they may not be able to continue their jobs, such as truck drivers, pilots, military personnel, or those with other commercial licenses. Patients need to understand that the insulin is needed now because of the high glucose levels, but, once in control, they may be able to try pills or some of the newer types of medications.[5]

Consult the dietitian as soon as possible; to assist and answer those questions facilitates the many other things that need to be learned. Carbohydrate-counting meal planning is the standard for persons with type 1 or 2 diabetes, but may not be the best plan in the beginning. It can be intimidating and confusing to start with. It also takes someone who is willing to do daily food logs for close evaluation at follow-up.[5] Keep things simple for new patients, unless they have read about it and ask. Internet resources are abundant, but recommend reputable sites.

One study explored patients' perceptions about barriers to their self-management, to help explain the poor health outcomes among minority patients. They included 31 predominately African American patients with diabetes, using open-ended questions about knowledge of current health status, medication use, continuity of care, blood glucose level, and nutrition. The primary barrier to diabetes self-management resulted from lack of knowledge of target blood glucose and blood pressure. This study identified new concerns that could be associated with poor health outcomes among minority patients because variations were attributed to the individual's knowledge and opinions rather than the patient's age, sex, or culture. Also, some of the participants found some of the health information to be confusing.[15] The limited health literacy seen in this study could help explain several of the barriers to self-management.

In 2008, a study by Lippa and Klein[16] identified that most participants failed to adequately understand the disease, typically because they were overwhelmed by or misunderstood rule-based instructions. Understanding of the dynamics underlying glucose regulation was also critical for effective self-management. They concluded that diabetes education needed to include the dynamics underlying self-management and to emphasize problem-solving and decision-making skills.[16]

WHY?

When a person is first diagnosed with diabetes or prediabetes, the earlier control is begun, the better. Education takes time, and patients' glucose control depends on how well they understand the who, what, when, where, and whys of their new lifestyle. Behavior changes will be ongoing over the next month to years. Beginning as soon as possible, introducing the new terms and explanations of how their body works is essential. A position statement, *Management of Hyperglycemia in Type 2 diabetes: a Patient-centered Approach*, by the American Diabetes Association (ADA) and the European Association for the Study of Diabetes (EASD) supports starting from diagnosis. Also, they recommend that patients have a say from the beginning in what their goals should be and what they want, focusing more on patient-centered care than on an algorithm of medications, as was previously done by other groups' recommendations and reviews. They recommend consideration of several factors (duration of disease, life expectancy, significance of cardiovascular disease, history of hypoglycemia, extensive comorbid conditions, advanced complications) to determine the glucose and HbA1C goals.[8]

Evidence indicates that a self-management program based on improving self-efficacy in managing diabetes can reduce the risk of a further cardiac event. In 2009, a pilot program using an experimental design was done in Brisbane, Australia, to develop a cardiac-diabetes self-management program (CDSMP). The results showed the feasibility of the CDSMP for patients with type 2 diabetes in critical care units in their transition to home.[17]

The 2012 ADA Standards of Medical Care recommend HbA1C of less than 7.0% to reduce the incidence of microvascular disease (eyes, kidneys). They also think that is it reasonable to suggest more stringent HbA1C goals (such as <6.5%) if they can be achieved without significant hypoglycemia or other adverse effects of treatment. They suggest that appropriate patients for this tighter control include those with short duration of diabetes, long life expectancy, and no significant cardiovascular disease. Less stringent HbA1C goals, such as less than 8.0%, may be appropriate for patients with a history of severe hypoglycemia, limited life expectancy, advanced microvascular or macrovascular complications, extensive comorbid conditions, or those with longstanding diabetes in whom the general goal is difficult to attain despite appropriate glucose monitoring and self-management skills and effective doses of multiple glucose-lowering agents, including insulin.[5,8,9] The landmark study, the Diabetes Control and Complications Trial (DCCT), showed that persons with type 1 diabetes who were recently diagnosed and started on intensive glycemic control were associated with significantly decreased rates of microvascular (retinopathy, nephropathy) and neuropathic complications.[18] Early intensive glycemic control has been shown to decrease long-term rates of microvascular and neuropathic complications in patients with type 2 diabetes.[19,20]

Intensive control usually means basal and bolus insulin doses, or 4 to 5 insulin injections. Many patients are shocked simply to learn that they have a new disease, without the need to do several injections. Many people will not know what questions to ask. Referral to a diabetes education program is recommended before discharge, to ensure that patients have the skills to maintain their glucose control, and to learn about the other areas that are also important. They also need to have a physician or group that will see them soon after discharge to evaluate their glucose log. They also need to know who to call if their glucose levels suddenly spike back up. Understanding the symptoms of infection is also important before they are discharged. Early recognition of any complication means earlier treatment. Help patients to understand that, when their glucose levels stay increased after a period of good control, it can indicate a hidden infection, such as urinary, dental, or sinus infections. They need to have a doctor or provider to call to discuss any symptoms or problems.

SUMMARY

The incidence of patients hospitalized with diabetes and hyperglycemia continues to increase, requiring early education and skills before their discharge. Studies are confirming that adequate education decreases their initial and long-term risks for acute and chronic complications, readmissions, and extended length of stay. These patients should be identified early by evaluating glucose and HbA1C levels of patients with steroids, infection, sepsis, wounds, high blood pressure, or known diabetes. Initiating education early, and coordination with other health care members, enhances learning, coordination with transfer, and optimal discharge. Critical care nurses need to be involved, starting with basic education about diabetes, symptoms, causes and treatment of these symptoms, monitoring, insulin, injections, goals for glucose levels, prevention of infection, and the balance of food, diet, medication, and exercise. If diabetic ketoacidosis is involved, additional education is needed about type 1 diabetes, symptoms of diabetic ketoacidosis, and possible causes (even if not newly diagnosed), prevention of future episodes, adequate testing for glucose and acetone when ill, adequate hydration, and sick day management. Early referral to a diabetes educator is essential, if available in the hospital. Dietitian referral while in the hospital is recommended. Follow-up referral for a diabetes self-management program should be provided. Allow patients to express questions, their current understanding of the disease, what symptoms they have, whether they have been testing glucose levels at home, and if not, why not? Are they willing to start? What do they think is the most challenging change that they need to make? The family or significant others should be involved with all education, too. Having booklets and Web site information readily available helps them understand the scope of changes that usually need to be made. They can then bring their questions back to discuss with someone within the health care team, to ensure that they understand what the patient's initial goals may be, what follow-up will be needed, and who and when to call if their glucose levels do not stabilize.

ACKNOWLEDGMENTS

I would like to acknowledge MD Anderson Cancer Center Endocrinology Service team for supporting me to assist our patients with understanding their diabetes, treatment plans, and goals. These people are: Victor Lavis, MD; Celia Levesque, RN, CNS, CDE, BC-ADM, FNP; Veronica Brady, RN, FNP; Kathleen Crawford, ANP; Ashley Martin, FNP; and Johnny Rollins, FNP.

REFERENCES

1. Donihi AC, Raval D, Saul M, et al. Prevalence and predictors of corticosteroid-related hyperglycemia in hospitalized patients. Endocr Pract 2006;12(4):358–62.
2. Centers for Disease Control and Prevention. 2011 National Diabetes Fact Sheet. 2011. Available at: http://www.cdc.gov/diabetes/pubs/estimates11htm. Accessed June 1, 2012.

3. Saberi F, Heyland D, Lam M, et al. Prevalence, incidence, and clinical resolution of insulin resistance in critically ill patients: an observational study. JPEN J Parenter Enteral Nutr 2008;32:227.
4. McCowen KC, Malhotra A, Bistrian BR. Stress-induced hyperglycemia. Crit Care Clin 2001;17:107.
5. American Diabetes Association. Standards of medical care in diabetes-2012. Diabetes Care 2012;35(Suppl 1):S11–63.
6. Umpierrez GE, Kitabchi AE. Diabetic ketoacidosis: risk factors and management strategies. Treat Endocrinol 2003;2:95–108.
7. Department of Health and Human Service' National Diabetes Education Program and National Institutes of Health NIH Publication No 09-4343 Rev April 2009. Available at: www.YourDiabetesInfo.org. Accessed June 1, 2012.
8. Inzucchi SE, Bergenstal RM, Buse JB, et al. Management of hyperglycemia in type 2 diabetes: a patient-centered approach. Position statement of the American Diabetes Association and the European Association for the Study of Diabetes. Diabetes Care 2012;35:1364–79.
9. American Association of Diabetes Educators. AADE7: measurable behavior change is the desired outcome of diabetes education. Available at: http://www.diabeteseducator.org/ProfessionalResources/AADE7/Background.html. Accessed June 1, 2012.
10. Morrison M. Post-pancreatic resection: general overview and unique complications. Dimens Crit Care Nurs 2010;29:157–62.
11. Haas L, Maryniuk M, Beck J, et al. National standards for diabetes self-management education and support. Diabetes Educ 2012;38:619–23.
12. Stetson B, Schlundt D, Payrot M, et al. Monitoring in diabetes self-management: issues and recommendations for improvement. Popul Health Manag 2011;14: 189–97.
13. Wild D, von Maltzahn R, Brohan E, et al. A critical review of the literature on fear on hypoglycemia in diabetes: implications for diabetes management and patient education. Patient Educ Couns 2007;68:10–5.
14. Pollom RK, Pollom RD. Utilization of a multidisciplinary team for inpatient diabetes care. Crit Care Nurs Q 2004;27:185–8.
15. Onwudiwe NC, Mullins CD. Barriers to self-management of diabetes: a qualitative study among low-income minority diabetics. Ethn Dis 2011;21:27–32.
16. Lippa KD, Klein HA. Portraits of patient cognition: how patients understand diabetes self-care. Can J Nurs Res 2008;40:80–95.
17. Wu CJ, Chang AM, McDowell J. Innovative self-management programme for diabetics following coronary care unit admission. Int Nurs Rev 2009;56:396–9.
18. The Diabetes Control and Complications Trial Research Group. The effect of intensive treatment of diabetes on the development and progression of long-term complications in insulin-dependent diabetes mellitus. N Engl J Med 1993; 329:977–86.
19. Ohkubo Y, Kishikawa H, Araki E, et al. Intensive insulin therapy prevents the progression of diabetic microvascular complications in Japanese patients with non-insulin-dependent diabetes mellitus: a randomized prospective 6-year study. Diabetes Res Clin Pract 1995;28:103–17.
20. UK prospective diabetes study (UKPDS) group. Effect of intensive blood-glucose control with metformin on complications in overweight patients with type 2 diabetes (UKPDS 34). Lancet 1993;352:854–65.

Limb Salvage for Veterans with Diabetes

To Care for Him Who Has Borne the Battle

Linda Wills Gibson, RN, MSN, CRRN, ANP-C*,
Ashraf Abbas, RN, MSN, ACNP-BC

KEYWORDS

- Diabetes • Diabetic foot ulcer • Amputation • Veterans Administration Hospital
- Limb salvage program

KEY POINTS

- Diabetes is the leading cause of nontraumatic lower limb amputation.
- Many lower limb amputations could have been prevented through a combination of diabetes control and foot care.
- The Veterans Administration Hospital in Houston, Texas has a comprehensive program to help veterans prevent the loss of lower limbs and also to help rehabilitate patients after amputation.

INTRODUCTION

The incidence of diabetes mellitus worldwide has reached almost epidemic proportions, with nearly 26 million people affected by the disease in the United States alone.[1,2] Among US residents ages 65 years and older, 9 million or 26.9%, had diabetes in 2010. In 2005 to 2008, based on a fasting glucose of 100 to 125 mg/dL or a HbA1c level of 5.7% to 6.4%, 35% of US adults ages 20 years or older had prediabetes. Prediabetes is found in 50% of Americans older than 65. Applying this percentage to the entire US population in 2010 yields an estimated 79 million American adults ages 20 years or older with prediabetes.[1]

THE IMPACT OF DIABETES ON LOWER LIMB AMPUTATION

Diabetes is the leading cause of kidney failure, nontraumatic lower limb amputations, and new cases of blindness among adults in the United States. Diabetes is a major cause of heart disease and stroke, and is the seventh leading cause of death in the

Rehabilitation Care Line, Michael E. DeBakey Veterans Affairs Medical Center, 2002 Holcombe Boulevard, Houston, TX 77030, USA
* Corresponding author.
E-mail address: Linda.Gibson4@va.gov

Crit Care Nurs Clin N Am 25 (2013) 131–134
http://dx.doi.org/10.1016/j.ccell.2012.11.004
0899-5885/13/$ – see front matter Published by Elsevier Inc.

United States.[1] Along with this increased incidence, there has been a significant rise in other comorbidities commonly seen in patients with diabetes.[3] Ulcerations can have potential devastating complications because they cause up to 90% of the lower extremity amputations in patients with diabetes.[2] Many factors are involved in the decreased healing potential of a diabetic foot, all of which stem from the metabolic disorders associated with diabetes. The most important of these factors include level of uncontrolled hyperglycemia, reduced circulation and arterial flow, nutrition status, inability to offload the affected region of the foot, and the presence of infection. Even with advances in the medical and surgical management of diabetes, the 5-year rate of mortality remains poor at approximately 66% after amputation of a leg—a testament to the debilitating and morbid nature of diabetes.[2]

COST OF LOWER LIMB AMPUTATIONS IN PATIENTS WITH DIABETES

Diabetes mellitus complications are estimated to account for 13% of medical expenses, with annual costs reaching $26 billion. Lower limb ulceration is a well-recognized complication of diabetes mellitus, affecting 15% of all persons with the disease during their lifetime. Although most veterans will successfully heal their ulcers, lower limb amputation (LLA) will be performed on 15% to 20%. The inpatient cost of a single LLA exceeds $25,000, and there are additional outpatient expenses for physical therapy and follow-up care, including prosthetic limbs. Amputations have tremendous functional and psychological impact. Activity limitation is observed in 81% of persons with LLA. It is estimated that more than 50% of LLAs due to diabetes could have been prevented by timely intervention. To achieve this goal, a comprehensive management strategy of foot care for high-risk veterans is needed.[3]

PREVENTION OF LOWER LIMB AMPUTATIONS AT MICHAEL E DEBAKEY AT VA IN HOUSTON, TEXAS

Diabetic foot wounds are a serious matter at Michael E DeBakey VA, Houston, Texas. There are many reasons for this statement. Two of the main reasons are that our soldiers and their families should not suffer the trauma of amputation from diabetic foot ulcers. Second, the financial cost for treating diabetic ulcers, amputations, and ongoing care after amputations is staggering. At DeBakey, physicians request therapy for their hospitalized patients and outpatients through the Rehabilitation Care Line. As rehabilitation nurse practitioners, the authors obtain a history and physical examination on veterans and write therapy orders if indicated. When the authors write therapy orders for a soldier who has had an amputation, their chart usually contains 2 to 3 months of records of treatment and surgical procedures before the amputation became the only remaining choice. Sometimes, the soldier would say that he or she was not careful enough or did not seek medical attention fast enough to avoid amputation. On one occasion, a soldier with a below-the-knee amputation stated "it was my fault; I was fishing and stepped on a fish hook; I didn't go to the doctor and my foot got infected."

To avoid negative outcomes like the one mentioned above, the Veterans Administration (VA) established a national program called Prevention of Amputation for Veterans Everywhere (PAVE). The purpose of the program is to identify and provide care to veterans at risk for limb loss and who have developed foot or leg problems that could predispose them to possible limb loss. Risk referral criteria include patients with a history of diabetes, progressive peripheral neuropathy, peripheral vascular disease, tobacco abuse, impaired lower extremity sensation, lower extremity ulcers, prior amputation, absent lower extremity pulses, pressure points, and claudication.[4]

Multiple services for lower extremity evaluation include; patient education, ambulating aids, assistive devices, contact source for questions and problems, referral to specialty clinics based on medical need, diabetes education, podiatry, endocrinology, smoking cessation, vascular surgery, prosthetics, orthotics, orthopedics, physical medicine and rehabilitation, nutrition service, low vision services, Telehealth, and Telemove programs.[4]

At DeBakey, PAVE education classes are offered for low risk and moderate risk patients with diabetes. High-risk patients with diabetes are evaluated in individual clinic visits. All patients are educated on laboratory values including HbA1c, blood glucose, and cholesterol. The importance of taking medicine as ordered, diabetes diet compliance, and 30 minutes of exercise 5 days per week, especially walking, are discussed and strongly recommended. Groups are lively and veterans are encouraged to talk about health concerns and ask questions. Family members are welcome in class and at individual appointments.

A thorough history and physical, including foot examination, are performed on high-risk patients with diabetes during individual clinic visits. The lower extremity examination includes ankle brachial index, foot temperature, O_2 saturation, and monofilament check for loss of protective sensation. Foot pulses are palpated and examined with Doppler ultrasound if pulses are not felt. Immediate action is taken for severe vascular compromise or wounds that place the patient at risk for limb loss.

Veterans in PAVE are urged to seek prompt medical care for extremity injuries, infected wounds or decreased circulation. Veterans are educated on how positive lifestyle choices, such as diet compliance, tobacco cessation, and consistent exercise, can make a positive impact on the quality of their lives. High-risk patients with diabetes can be referred to the Health Buddy outpatient program. In this program, a computer unit (Health Buddy) is attached to a veteran's home phone or computer. Veterans receive a blood pressure cuff and weight scale. This computer unit allows VA registered nurses to monitor glucose, vital signs, laboratory work, and weight, and educate or assist the veteran to lower their glucose/HbA1c levels. Patients are usually referred to the PAVE clinic by their providers. Many patients referred to this clinic have diabetes with elevated HbA1c and blood glucose. Obesity, hypertension, osteoarthritis, hyperlipidemia, strokes, cardiac problems, renal failure, and lower extremity amputations are often present.

If a patient has neuropathy with a loss of protection sensation, the patient is instructed on the prevention of foot injury. Home safety, such as removing rugs, using nightlights, and wearing shoes to avoid falls and to protect the feet, is stressed. Prosthetics may be consulted for diabetic shoes for patients to prevent foot injury. Blood glucose meters and supplies are provided for all veterans who use insulin. The Managing overweight and/or Obesity for Veterans Everywhere (MOVE) program for weight management and heart healthy eating classes are held twice monthly at the VA I Houston, Texas. Also, a walk-in/no appointment dietitian clinic is available all day throughout the week for diet issues. These issues may include weight loss, diabetes, lowering blood pressure, kidney disease, side effects of cancer treatment, gastrointestinal problems, home tube feeding, weight gain, and many others. Dietary counseling is available in Houston as well as other locations.

Multiple therapies for rehabilitation are available including physical, occupational, kinetic, and pool therapy. The VA pharmacy representative will meet with the veteran and educate them on the action and side effects of the medication. In addition, mental health services may be consulted for providers, support groups, and psychotherapy. Because the VA provides comprehensive and ongoing care, all referrals can be taken care of within the system and results will be recorded in the patient's electronic medical record. Any referring provider will be aware when the patient is scheduled for various clinics and the result of those visits. This referral helps to ensure continuity of comprehensive care.[4] Finally, a limb salvage program has been established at DeBakey by the Vascular Surgery Service. This rapid response team may be paged by any provider at the VA and will respond immediately 24 hours a day 7 days a week to concerns. Patients are triaged; acute wounds or decreased circulation will be addressed immediately, and the patient will be hospitalized for emergency care. Nonemergent conditions may be transported to the vascular surgery area for care or testing or referred to other clinics as appropriate.[5]

A limb salvage meeting is held monthly and includes infectious disease specialists, podiatrists, orthopedic surgeons, vascular surgeons, nurses, nurse practitioners, and physical therapists. A variety of subjects related to wound care and treatment are discussed at meetings. Often members present specific case studies of non-healing wounds and request input from other disciplines. Education for groups of veterans with nurse practitioners giving limb salvage prevention information is planned. The Limb Salvage program is new and challenging and gives information and support to all disciplines. Because it is known that diabetic wounds with poor circulation worsen rapidly, limbs are being saved daily by the rapid response of the Limb Salvage Service at Michael E DeBakey VA, Houston, Texas.[6]

REFERENCES

1. Centers for Disease Control and Prevention. National diabetes fact sheet: National estimates and general information on diabetes and prediabetes in the United States 2011. Available at: http://www.cdc.gov/diabetes/pubs/factsheet11.htm. Accessed September 1, 2012.
2. Hsu A. Diabetic foot ulcer 2012. Available at: http://www.orthopaedia.net/display/Main/Diabetic+foot+ulcer. Accessed September 1, 2012.
3. Fotieo G, Reiber G, Carter J, et al. Diabetic amputations in the VA: are there opportunities for interventions? J Rehabil Res Dev 1999;36:55–9.
4. Department of Veterans Affairs Veterans Health Administration. VHA Directive 2012-020 Prevention of amputations in veterans everywhere (PAVE) program. Available at: http://www.va.gov/vhapublications/ViewPublication.asp?pub_ID=2778. Accessed September 1, 2012.
5. Fitzgerald R, Mills J, Joseph W, et al. The diabetic rapid response acute foot team: 7 essential skills for targeted limb salvage. Eplasty 2009. Available at: http://www.ncbi.nlm.nih.gov/pmc/articles/PMC2680239/. Accessed September 1, 2012.
6. Iorio MI, Goldstein J, Adams M, et al. Functional Limb Salvage in the Diabetic Patient: The Use of a Collagen Bilayer Matrix and Risk Factors for Amputation. Plast Reconstr Surg 2011 Jan;127(1):260–7.

Index

Note: Page numbers of article titles are in **boldface** type.

A

ACCORD (Action to Control Cardiovascular Disease and Diabestes), blood pressure goal, 74
ACEIs (Angiotensin-converting enzyme inhibitors), 77–79
ADVANCE (Action in Diabetes and Vascular Disease: Preterax and Diamicrom MR controlled Evaluation), blood pressure goal, 74
alpha-Adrenoceptor antagonists, 88–89
alpha-Glucosidase inhibitor(s), acarbose, 44
   miglitol, 44
Amylin agonists, pramlintide, 47
Angiotensin-converting enzyme inhibitors (ACEIs), 77–79
Angiotensin receptor blockers (ARBs), 87–88
Antidiabetic medications, noninsulin, in hospitalized patients, **39–53**
Antihypertensive medication(s), ACEIs, 77–79
   alpha-adrenoceptor antagonists, 88–89
   and associated drug classes, 80–86
   ARBs, 79
   beta-blockers, 87–88
   calcium channel blockers, 87–88
   diuretics, 86–87
   nitrodilators, 89
   potassium channel openers, 89
   renin inhibitors, 90
   selection of monotherapy *vs.* combination therapy, 76–77
     recommendations for initial, 77
   sympatholytics, centrally acting, 89
   tests before starting, 75–76, 78–79
   vasodilators, direct-acting, 89
ARBs (Angiotensin receptor blockers), 87–88

B

beta Blockers, 87–88
Biguanide(s), metformin, 43–44
   perioperative use of, 23–24, 27
Blood pressure, accurate measurement of, 73
   goal for, ACCORD, 74
     ADVANCE, 74
     INVEST, 75

Crit Care Nurs Clin N Am 25 (2013) 135–141
http://dx.doi.org/10.1016/S0899-5885(12)00118-9
0899-5885/13/$ – see front matter © 2013 Elsevier Inc. All rights reserved.

ccnursing.theclinics.com

Moving?

Make sure your subscription moves with you!

To notify us of your new address, find your **Clinics Account Number** (located on your mailing label above your name), and contact customer service at:

Email: journalscustomerservice-usa@elsevier.com

800-654-2452 (subscribers in the U.S. & Canada)
314-447-8871 (subscribers outside of the U.S. & Canada)

Fax number: 314-447-8029

Elsevier Health Sciences Division
Subscription Customer Service
3251 Riverport Lane
Maryland Heights, MO 63043

*To ensure uninterrupted delivery of your subscription, please notify us at least 4 weeks in advance of move.

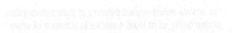